Oral Health for an Ageing Population

Evidence, Policy, Practice and Evaluation

Kakuhiro Fukai
Fukai Institute of Health Science
3-86 Hikonari Misato-shi
Saitama
Japan, 341-0003

WILEY Blackwell

Registered Offices
John Wiley & Sons, Inc., 111 River Street, Hoboken, NJ 07030, USA
John Wiley & Sons Ltd, The Atrium, Southern Gate, Chichester, West Sussex, PO19 8SQ, UK

For details of our global editorial offices, customer services, and more information about Wiley products visit us at www.wiley.com.

Wiley also publishes its books in a variety of electronic formats and by print-on-demand. Some content that appears in standard print versions of this book may not be available in other formats.

Limit of Liability/Disclaimer of Warranty
The contents of this work are intended to further general scientific research, understanding, and discussion only and are not intended and should not be relied upon as recommending or promoting scientific method, diagnosis, or treatment by physicians for any particular patient. In view of ongoing research, equipment modifications, changes in governmental regulations, and the constant flow of information relating to the use of medicines, equipment, and devices, the reader is urged to review and evaluate the information provided in the package insert or instructions for each medicine, equipment, or device for, among other things, any changes in the instructions or indication of usage and for added warnings and precautions. While the publisher and authors have used their best efforts in preparing this work, they make no representations or warranties with respect to the accuracy or completeness of the contents of this work and specifically disclaim all warranties, including without limitation any implied warranties of merchantability or fitness for a particular purpose. No warranty may be created or extended by sales representatives, written sales materials or promotional statements for this work. This work is sold with the understanding that the publisher is not engaged in rendering professional services. The advice and strategies contained herein may not be suitable for your situation. You should consult with a specialist where appropriate. The fact that an organization, website, or product is referred to in this work as a citation and/or potential source of further information does not mean that the publisher and authors endorse the information or services the organization, website, or product may provide or recommendations it may make. Further, readers should be aware that websites listed in this work may have changed or disappeared between when this work was written and when it is read. Neither the publisher nor authors shall be liable for any loss of profit or any other commercial damages, including but not limited to special, incidental, consequential, or other damages.

Library of Congress Cataloging-in-Publication Data
Names: Fukai, Kakuhiro, author.
Title: Oral health for an ageing population : evidence, policy, practice and evaluation / Kakuhiro Fukai.
Description: Hoboken, NJ : Wiley-Blackwell, 2025. | Includes bibliographical references and index.
Identifiers: LCCN 2024031449 (print) | LCCN 2024031450 (ebook) | ISBN 9781119541264 (paperback) | ISBN 9781119541295 (adobe pdf) | ISBN 9781119541271 (epub)
Subjects: MESH: Oral Health | Aged | Health Policy
Classification: LCC RK55.A3 (print) | LCC RK55.A3 (ebook) | NLM WU 113 | DDC 617.6/010846–dc23/eng/20240801
LC record available at https://lccn.loc.gov/2024031449
LC ebook record available at https://lccn.loc.gov/2024031450

Cover Design: Wiley
Cover Image: © adamkaz/Getty Images

Set in 9.5/12.5pt STIXTwoText by Straive, Pondicherry, India

Printed in Singapore
M093341_071124

Contents

Preface

Over the past decade, it has become clearer and clearer to me that more attention and research is needed globally at the intersection of population ageing and oral health, and indeed, awareness of the importance of this issue is now higher than ever. At both the national and international level, oral health throughout the life course is now seen as a fundamental and essential component of socioeconomic development. In 2015, I helped organize the 2015 World Congress on Oral Health and Ageing, which was held jointly by the Japan Dental Association and the World Health Organization in Tokyo, Japan, where the "Tokyo Declaration on Dental Care and Oral Health for Healthy Longevity" was issued. I then began serving as chair of the World Dental Federation's (FDI) Oral Health for an Ageing Population (OHAP) task team, a role that has continued to this day. It was at the 2017 FDI World Congress in Madrid, Spain that the idea for this book was hatched.

The purpose of the OHAP task team was to build on the success of the 2015 Tokyo Declaration, engaging in further discussions and collaboration with colleagues around the world to put the goals of the declaration into practice. Phase I of the project concluded in 2020 and Phase II began in 2021, leading to the development and provision of education and policy recommendations to dental associations, government officials and dental professionals in Europe, North America and South America. Phase III started in 2024, with the goal of promoting the implementation of oral health campaigns and projects in all regions of the world, regardless of development level. I have also personally visited a number of Asian countries, as part of Japanese government assistance efforts, to discuss the topic of "Dental and Oral Health Care in Ageing Societies" with government officials and dental professionals, and to make recommendations based on Japan's experiences. Furthermore, I have visited Nepal for two weeks nearly every year for the past three decades as part of an NGO to implement community health programs for schools, mothers and children, and older persons, and to conduct community health worker training. Throughout all of these activities and roles, I have noticed that population ageing and oral health have become more and more important as economies develop and population ageing progresses. Even in low- and middle-income countries, there is a growing understanding that they will soon face the same ageing-related public health challenges that high-income countries are facing now.

In 2019, at the UN High-Level Meeting (HLM), it was determined that oral health would be included in the definition of Universal Health Coverage (UHC), which had already been established as one of the common global Sustainable Development Goals (SDGs). In a further sign of global attention on oral health issues, the 2021 WHO General Assembly adopted a resolution on oral health for the first time in 17 years.

Ageing has already been progressing rapidly in high-income nations, and it will soon begin to affect low- and middle-income nations as well. Meanwhile, the global burden of oral disease remains heavy, and health inequality remains an urgent global issue. The need for new, creative, and economically efficient solutions for achieving healthy longevity is therefore universal, but the health care system of each country and community must be uniquely tailored to its own circumstances. Evidence is accumulating that oral health plays an important role in general health, but this knowledge has not been effectively translated into policy and practice on a global scale. As researchers, health professionals, and policymakers in each country strive to move forward in this process, the lessons Japan has learned as a frontrunner in the field of public policy for an ageing society can provide insight and inspiration for other countries.

Japan was one of the first countries to implement a UHC system, and the system has been functioning successfully for more than 60 years. Japan was also the first country to be confronted with the challenges of a super-ageing society. For these reasons, Japan is currently engaged in an intensive process of making its healthcare system even more efficient, economical and prevention-oriented, with an eye to creating an ageing-friendly society. To achieve this, we are also trying to achieve more efficient and effective communication and collaboration among healthcare professionals in different fields.

There are many other examples of how countries around the world are dealing with these issues, with varying degrees of success. In the end, each country will need to find locally relevant and sustainable solutions to the problem of UHC. But in order to do so, we need to learn from each other's successes and failures, and above all we need to have access to the most current and applicable evidence.

The processes of assessing national and regional oral healthcare policies and sharing outcomes globally, addressing issues at both the global and national level, and identifying solutions for the future can only proceed efficiently if it is based on collaboration between professionals in all related fields and around the world. This book is, therefore, intended to help raise the awareness of not only dental clinicians but also a wide array of health professionals and policymakers regarding oral health for an ageing population. It will provide them with the evidence as well as the practical solutions they need to implement effective policies and practices. But perhaps even more important than current policymakers and practitioners, my sincere hope is that the information in this book will be taught in healthcare and health policy-related courses at the graduate and even undergraduate level. The people who will change the world 30 years from now (when people age 60 and over will account for 40% of the world's population) must begin, as early as possible in their education, to develop a vision for the type of evidence-based health policy that will lead to achieving healthy longevity globally. Evidence, public health policy, healthcare practices, and evaluation of the effectiveness of those practices are often studied as separate subjects and in abstract ways, but this book attempts to present them as elements of a connected and unified cycle that takes place in real-world situations in each country, where limited resources require hard choices.

Population ageing is by no means unique to high-income countries; it is an unavoidable fact for all humans that the risk of disease and disability increases with age. However, establishing and funding systems to maintain the health of older persons, including preventing oral diseases and oral function decline, is no easy task. It requires long-term, sustained effort and investment to resolve the significant and unique challenges faced by each country, which often include the financial burden, lack of an existing healthcare system on which to build, and lack of trained professionals. No matter the current political or economic situation, however, every nation should begin taking practical and strategic steps to provide access to oral health care services for all residents. Oral health must be seen as a basic human right for people of all ages, including older persons. After all, everyone has the right to speak, eat and laugh.

The process of researching and writing this book took longer than expected due to the COVID-19 pandemic, an unprecedented global public health crisis which began in January 2020. During this pandemic, older people were identified as a vulnerable population at higher risk of contracting the disease due to both ageing itself and the underlying respiratory and cardiovascular diseases that are associated with ageing. Indeed, elderly people experienced severe illness and death due to COVID-19 at a much higher rate than the general population during this period. On the other hand, recent research has reported that the maintenance of healthy oral status, including the prevention of periodontal disease, is associated with reduced severity of COVID-19 symptoms. The accumulation of oral health throughout the life course is reflected in the oral health and general health of older people. Provision of sufficient oral health services for the elderly population will also be key to dealing with future unexpected health crises similar to COVID-19.

The six chapters in this publication discuss the policy, practice and evaluation of oral health for an ageing population. This section provides a summary of each chapter.

Chapter 1. Global ageing and health
The unavoidable reality of population ageing is affecting our society on a global scale. Biological ageing makes older adults susceptible to disease and leads to a decline in the bodily functions needed for daily living. Dental and oral health are essential for the lifelong maintenance of quality of life (QOL), and research has also shown that they contribute to the maintenance and improvement of general health. As a matter of basic human rights, the goal of every society should be to provide high-quality dental care and oral health services to all residents and at all stages of life, especially for its most vulnerable populations, such as older adults and those with disabilities.

Life expectancy trends from 1950 to the end of the 21st century reveal an expected narrowing of the gap between the region with the lowest life expectancy (Africa) and the regions with the highest life expectancy (North America, Europe, Oceania). This gap will narrow from 30 years to about 10 years during this period. It is also clear that all regions of the world will have achieved a life expectancy of over 80 years by the end of this century.

However, in order to realize healthy longevity in our society, we need to work toward the following four objectives: 1) to increase life expectancy and prevent early death, 2) to prevent people from requiring long-term care, 3) to slow the decline in daily living functions that accompanies ageing, and 4) to promote healthy behaviour from the early years of adulthood based on the life course approach.

Chapter 2. Achieving oral health among older adults: Community and clinical approaches
Oral diseases have a higher prevalence than systemic diseases. The oral health of older people is particularly affected by tooth loss, which results from the accumulation of dental caries and worsening periodontal disease throughout one's life. Even when not accompanied by tooth loss, dental caries and periodontal disease themselves are also significant health risks that negatively affect the quality of life of older people. In addition, age-related decline in the muscle strength of the tongue, orbicularis oculus, and the masticatory and swallowing muscles, together with reduced saliva, leads to a gradual decline in oral function. Prevention of such oral function decline is important in its own right, and it is also important for the prevention of frailty and for preventing and reducing dependence on long-term care, because undernutrition is associated with frailty in the elderly. The risk of oral diseases continues throughout all life stages, so dental professionals are likely to care for patients frequently, regularly, and over a long period of time. This means that dental professionals are uniquely positioned to notice small, gradual changes in the physical and mental condition, including the oral function, of older patients.

Assessment of oral health status in older people requires community-wide screening in addition to full dental examinations at dental clinics. If examinations at dental clinics are the only approach utilized, it is difficult to catch the beginning stages of reduced oral function in healthy people and take appropriate community and individual measures.

In order to prevent NCDs and frailty, which are highly associated with oral health, there is a need for communities and dental institutions to collaborate to implement public health programmes which include assessment and screening and are based on the principle of inter-professional cooperation and driven by national policy.

This chapter, therefore, focuses on the importance of cooperation between local communities and dental institutions within the larger national healthcare system, which itself must be built around a stable medical insurance system and long-term care insurance system.

In addition, cognitive function decline has become a major health challenge for ageing societies, so it is essential to consider how dental treatment and dental health guidance can be adapted specifically for people with dementia. This chapter therefore describes how dental treatment can be integrated into national dementia policies, with a particular focus on the emerging role of dental care in preventing cognitive decline.

Chapter 3. The link between systemic health and oral health

The maintenance of dental and oral health over a lifetime, as well as efforts to prevent tooth loss and to retain and/or recover oral function, contributes to the prevention and control of non-communicable diseases (NCDs), which cause death or result in conditions requiring long-term care. Dental and oral health maintenance also help to slow the senescence (ageing) process and promote healthy and independent longevity by improving diet and social function. To what extent does the scientific evidence accumulated thus far support these claims? This chapter represents a wide-ranging, comprehensive review of the evidence regarding the effects of dental care and oral health on the various factors that damage health. This review leads us to a greater recognition, understanding, and visualization of the relationship between oral health and whole-body health. The unambiguous conclusion is that we must reform our health care systems based on that recognition. This evidence can also be used as the basis for discussing, planning and implementing future research programs and agendas.

Chapter 4. Universal health coverage and effective health policy: Lessons from Japan

Barriers to oral health services, including dental care for older people, need to be removed in order to make these vital services accessible to all. This is in line with the philosophy of Universal Health Care (UHC), which is also reflected in the Sustainable Development Goals (SDGs), that everyone should have access to basic health services. Oral health is a key indicator of overall health in older age. Better integration of oral health care into the general health care system is required.

This chapter explains the definition and philosophy of UHC as well as how UHC achievement is assessed based on each country's circumstances and resources.

In addition, Japan is a country where dental care has been covered under the public health insurance system since 1961, and programmes for the prevention of decline in oral function are positioned within the long-term care insurance system. In addition, there is a publicly-financed system of dental health check-ups throughout infancy, childhood, adulthood and old age. Another unique aspect of Japan's approach is that measures to prevent dental diseases and oral function decline are included in national health policies such as those targeting frailty, dementia, and NCDs. For these reasons, in this chapter Japan is presented as an example of how to position dental health and dental care within an advanced, effective, stable UHC system.

Any national UHC system needs to take into account the financial burden and to make effective and efficient use of human resources in the health sector. Cross-sector collaboration is therefore required, and it is effective to include oral health programmes in overall health policy rather than having an isolated policy that is specific to dental and oral health. As health systems differ in each country, it is advisable to build on and make use of the strengths of each system and for countries to share and learn from each other's UHC initiatives. Access to essential oral health services throughout life is a fundamental human right that should be ensured in every region and in every country.

Chapter 5. Lessons from the United Kingdom, Europe, North America and Australia
One of the goals of Universal Health Coverage is to create a healthcare system to provide equal accessibility to affordable healthcare for all people. Barriers to healthcare accessibility directly cause deterioration of health, particularly for the elderly and other vulnerable groups. Ageing populations and slow economic growth are prompting most developed nations to reconsider their social security systems, particularly in the area of healthcare reform. Developed countries share some common challenges: how to provide all residents with equal access to a fair, sustainable healthcare system with limited financial resources.

This chapter reviews the medical health insurance systems of seven developed, Western nations: the UK, Sweden, Australia, Canada, France, German, and the US. The characteristics and challenges of these countries' public health insurance systems are summarized based on research reports and government records from 1995 to 2019. Some of these countries have government-funded or social insurance-type systems, while others rely primarily on private insurance. In terms of dental insurance coverage, the developed countries covered in this chapter run the gamut, with some providing government-funded dental insurance, some providing partial coverage, and some relying entirely on private insurance coverage. There is room for improvement in terms of providing dental care to a wider range of people without imposing undue financial burden.

Dental care is not covered or only partially covered in most of the developed nations discussed in this chapter, even though dental treatments often impose a heavy financial burden on patients. Public health insurance in the US only serves as the primary source of coverage for persons in limited age ranges and those who have certain socioeconomic characteristics. There is potential for improvement so that a wider range of people can receive higher-quality public health care with reduced financial burden.

Chapter 6. Health policy in Asia: Overview and Vision
Population ageing is progressing throughout the world, and Asia is no exception. Over the next 30 years, ageing will accelerate rapidly in Asian countries. On the other hand, total fertility rate (TFR) has fallen in many Asian countries. This means that governments must take a two-pronged policy approach, implementing both a social security system for the elderly and a childcare support system for young families at the same time. This poses an impossible financial burden on such governments.

This chapter represents a close examination of the health insurance systems of Asian countries, which have a large number of elderly people. The characteristics and challenges of the health insurance systems of ten Asian countries (China, India, Indonesia, South Korea, Malaysia, Philippines, Singapore, Thailand, Indonesia, and Vietnam) are summarized, with a specific focus on identifying the funding sources of the health insurance system in each country, based on research reports and government records from 2008 to 2018. It is necessary to develop country-specific variations of UHC, and this can best be accomplished by sharing information and incorporating the most useful aspects of each country's system.

UHC is one solution to this problem. However, there are a number of obstacles preventing many countries from achieving UHC. These include insufficient financial resources, shortage of medical and dental professionals as well as medication and facilities, and the tendency of the wealthy to enrol in private insurance plans. Therefore, it is necessary for each country to work toward achieving UHC in a way that fits with its own specific history and circumstances, while sharing information, advice and successful ideas with each other. This type of cooperation and information sharing can contribute to progress toward achieving UHC not only in Asian countries, but also globally.

I would like express my sincere gratitude to the editors at Wiley who have shepherded this project from beginning to end: Jessica Evans, Erica Judisch, Jayadivya Saiprasad, Tanya McMullin, Katherine King, Oliver Raj, Sreemol Manikandan, Adam Campbell, and Anitha Jasmine Stanley. Their support, assistance, prodding, and persistence was invaluable in bringing this project to fruition. I would also like to thank my research assistant, Sachiko Onai-Hayakawa, for her tireless and reliable work on the figures, tables, and references. Finally, I would like to thank Jeffrey Huffman for his diligence and encouragement in editing this book over the past six years. Without his help, this book could not have been completed.

22nd September 2024   *Kakuhiro Fukai*

1

Global ageing and health

1.1   Introduction

The unavoidable reality of population ageing is affecting our society on a global scale. Biological ageing makes older adults susceptible to disease and leads to a decline in the bodily functions needed for daily living. Dental and oral health are essential for the lifelong maintenance of quality of life (QOL), and research has also shown that they contribute to the maintenance and improvement of general health. As a matter of basic human rights, the goal of every society should be to provide high-quality dental care and oral health services to all residents and at all stages of life, especially for its most vulnerable populations, such as older adults and those with disabilities.

To ensure that dental care and oral health contribute to attaining healthy longevity, the accumulation of clear evidence must be prioritized, and action must be taken to secure and maintain the prominent role of dental care and oral health within an effective and efficient social security system and healthcare policy.

In that context, this chapter provides an overview of global ageing and global health, with special attention given to their relation to oral health.

1.2 Changes in the world population and longevity

The world population increased almost three-fold from 2.57 billion in 1950 to 8 billion in 2022 and is projected to reach 8.5 billion in 2030, 9.7 billion in 2050 and 10.4 billion in 2100. The greater portion of this population will be living in low and middle-income countries (LMICs; UN 2022) (Figure 1.1).

A historical survey of population ageing reveals that the average human life expectancy was about 40 years all the way up to the 18th century. As a result of decreases in infection-related deaths, life expectancy rose to 50 years from the 18th to the 20th century and then rose dramatically to 80 years from the middle of the 20th century to the present day (UN 2022) (Figure 1.2).

Figure 1.2 shows the estimated trends of life expectancy at birth in different regions of the world from 1950 to the end of this century. The clearest pattern here is the narrowing of the gap between the region with the lowest life expectancy (Africa) and the regions with the highest life expectancy (North America, Europe, Oceania). This gap narrows from 30 years to about 10 years during this period. It is also clear from this graph that all regions of the world will have achieved a life expectancy of over 80 years by the end of this century (UN 2019).

The percentage of older adults increased from 7.7% in 1950 to 16.1% in 2010 in the high-income countries and from 3.8% to 5.8% during the same time period in LMICs (UN 2022). Population ageing is occurring in all regions of the world and in countries at all income levels and is progressing at a faster rate in LMICs.

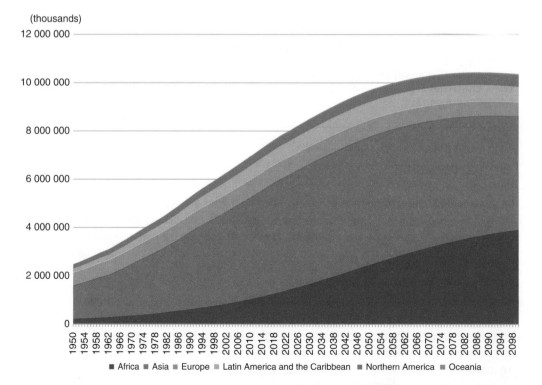

Figure 1.1 World population by major area, 1950–2100 (United Nations 2022).

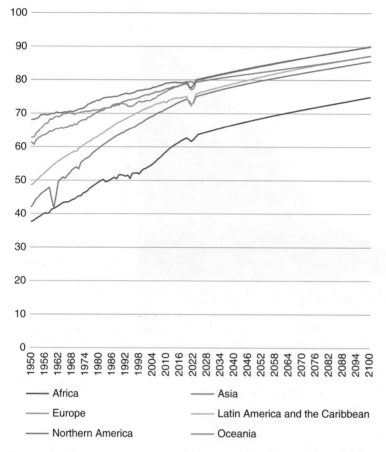

Figure 1.2 Life expectancy at birth (both sexes combined) by region, 1950–2100 (years) (UN 2022).

Looking at the same phenomenon from a different perspective, Figure 1.3 shows the total older adult population in each region (UN 2019). The percentage of older adults aged 65 years and over is also on the increase in each region (UN 2019) (Figure 1.4). This provides a visual representation of the fact that most of the older adults in the world live in Asia, and that trend will continue to increase, with the African older adult population following in the second half of the century. From the standpoint of global public health, if the goal is to ensure that no one or no region is left behind, improvement of healthcare provisions in Asia and Africa will have an outsized effect. Confronting this problem will require the sharing of experience, wisdom and evidence on a more massive and global scale than we have seen before now. Another important challenge will be to improve and increase data collection systems, needs assessment research and the implementation of public health programmes and systems in Asia and Africa, along with the evaluation thereof (including cost-effectiveness).

Living longer lives has long been a desire and goal of humans and human societies, and in the 20th century the world saw great increases in both population and longevity, largely due to scientific and medical advances, and the accompanying accumulation of knowledge, that have been achieved in each country. However, it is an unavoidable fact that ageing leads to a decline in the physical and mental functions needed for daily living, as well as increasing vulnerability to disease.

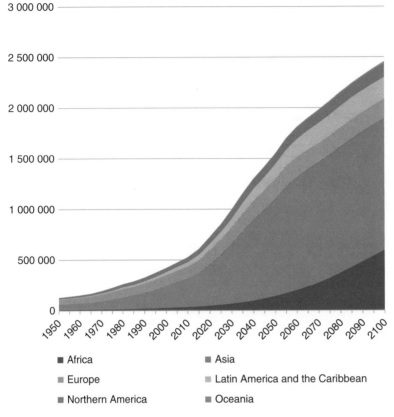

Figure 1.3 Population (both sexes combined) by 5-year age cohorts aged 65 years and over by region, 1950–2100 (thousands) (UN 2019).

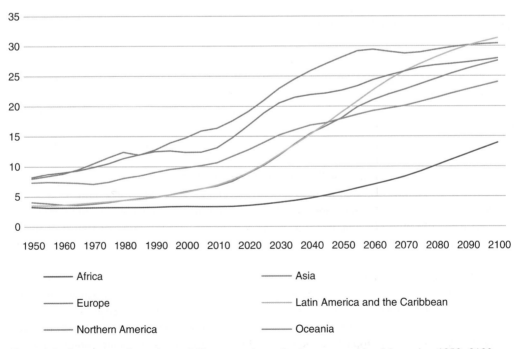

Figure 1.4 Percentage of people aged 65 years and over (both sexes combined) by region, 1950–2100 (United Nations 2022).

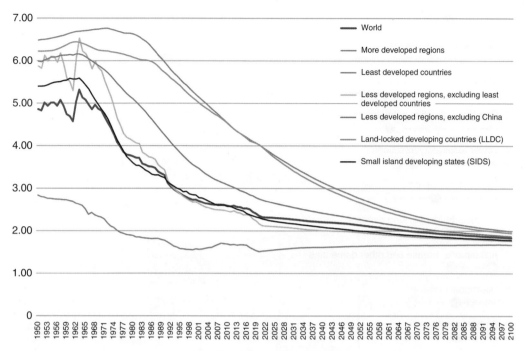

Figure 1.5   Total fertility by major area, 1950–2100 (children per woman) (UN 2022).

For this reason, many challenges still need to be addressed in order to achieve a society in which all older people can live with dignity and security. Such challenges include the establishment and maintenance of a sustainable social security system characterized by comprehensive healthcare provision, a system of long-term care provision, a solid financial resource basis for these services, and the continual accumulation of research.

In addition, while Asia and Africa still have relatively high fertility (Figure 1.5) that can, if used effectively, be viewed as a 'population bonus' (promoting economic development), these two regions will, in the second half of the century, follow the population dynamics trend that the developed world is currently experiencing – namely a 'population onus' where a decreasing working-age population must support an increasing ageing population. Therefore, as Asia and Africa begin developing their healthcare system, they must keep in mind the need for long-term financial sustainability, the keys to which are community-based, education-oriented, prevention-focused public health systems rather than after-the-fact medical and pharmacological treatment (UN 2022).

The world population is nearly 8 billion and rising, but the pace of increase is expected to slow over the next century, particularly in developed countries. As developing countries achieve greater economic development due to educational advancements and technological innovation, the rate of their population increase will slow down as well, eventually leading a more stable and sustainable global population.

1.3   Causes of death and determinants of life expectancy

Figure 1.6 shows the leading causes of death globally in 2020, and eight of the 10 leading causes of death are non-communicable diseases (NCDs). While acute diseases such as infections and diarrhoeal diseases remain the top causes of death in low-income countries, chronic diseases such as

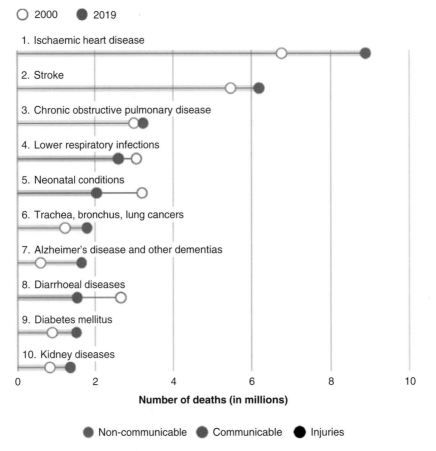

Figure 1.6 Leading causes of death globally (WHO 2020d).

ischaemic heart disease, stroke and cancer are the main causes of death in high-income countries [World Health Organization (WHO) 2020c].

As a country's economy improves, the mortality of pregnant women and newborns declines, but other challenges need to be overcome in order to continue extending life expectancy – in particular, the prevention of disease in the early years of adulthood (thereby reducing premature mortality) and the reduction of mortality in older adults. As a result, developing countries are facing the triple burden of acute infections, chronic diseases and newly emerging infections (Beard 2016) (Figure 1.7).

In Japan, for example, these diseases, such as cancer, heart disease, pneumonia and cerebrovascular disease, account for approximately 70% of all deaths [Ministry of Health Labour and Welfare (MHLW), Japan 2021a] (Figure 1.8). Theoretically, if these diseases can be successfully prevented (or at least become non-fatal), we can expect an extension in the average life expectancy of 3–4 years in the case of cancer, approximately 1.5 years in the case of heart disease, and around 1 year in the case of pneumonia and cerebrovascular diseases (MHLW of Japan 2021b) (Figure 1.9). This same strategy applies to LMICs as well, which over the past 50 years have been experiencing their own steady shift from infectious diseases to NCDs (WHO 2011).

Figure 1.10 shows the survival curve of the Japanese population. The number of deaths peaks at age 85 in men and age 91 in women (MHLW of Japan 2020a). The average life expectancy is

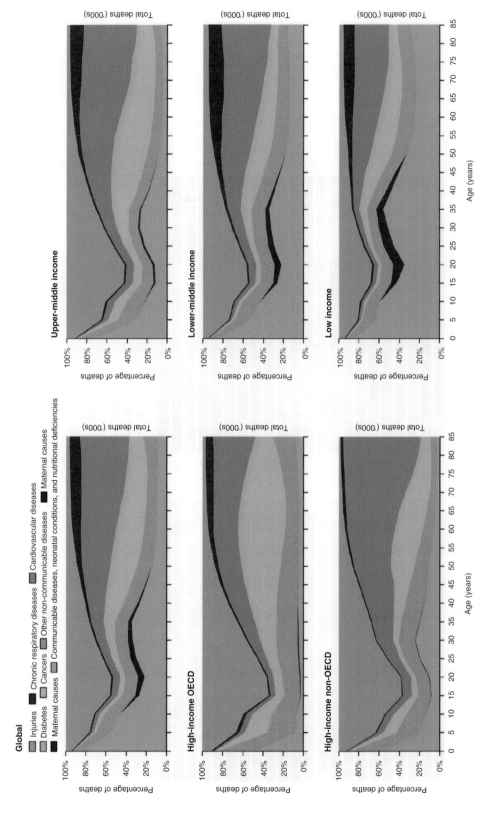

Figure 1.7 Mortality at different ages for countries of low, middle, and high income, 2012. *Source*: Beard, J.R. 2016/with permission of Elsevier.

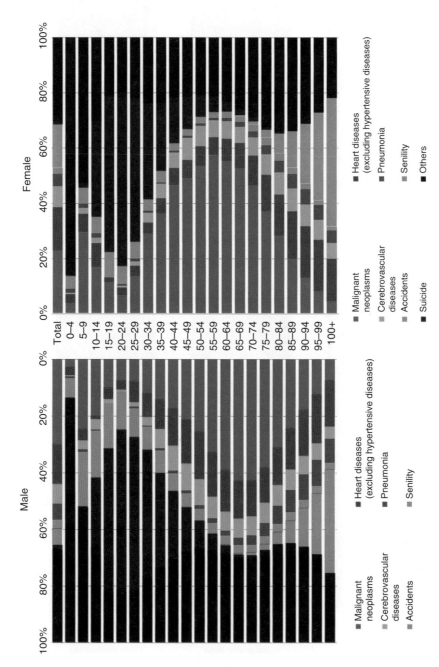

Figure 1.8 Proportion of leading cause of death by sex and age in Japan, 2021. *Source:* Ministry of Health, Labour and Welfare, Japan 2021, Vital Statics, 2021.

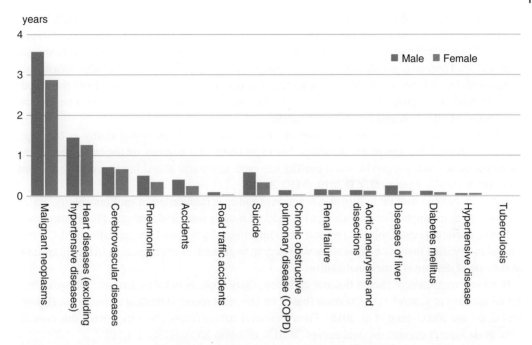

Figure 1.9 Estimated increase in life expectancy when specified causes of death are eliminated in Japan, 2020. *Source:* Ministry of Health, Labour and Welfare, Japan 2021, Life table, 2021.

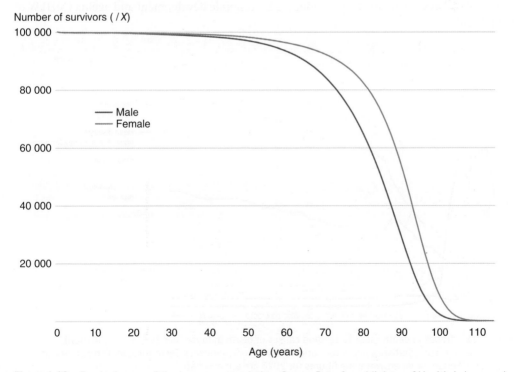

Figure 1.10 Survival curve of the Japanese population. *Source:* Data from Ministry of Health, Labour and Welfare of Japan (2020a), Life table.

81.6 years for men and 87.7 years for women, but what is not emphasized often enough is that the survival rate at that age is approximately 60% for both men and women (MHLW of Japan 2020b). The survival curve begins to decline from age 65, and then begins to decline more steeply from age 75. Therefore, *people are most likely to die between ages 75 and 100*. This also means that illness and dependence are at their peak within this age range. This means that, from the standpoint of healthcare provision, the period of life beyond the average life span should be the primary focus of attention and resource allocation.

All humans experience a certain degree of unavoidable loss of functional ability as they age, especially beyond the age of 65. Although life expectancy of a country or region is affected by socioeconomic level, the gap between healthy life expectancy and actual life expectancy remains constant at around 9 years (OECD 2019; WHO 2020a).

This unavoidable decline in intrinsic functional ability is manifested in multimorbidity, which consists of organ function decline along with reduced muscle mass and strength. That in turn leads to frailty, declining immunological resistance to infectious disease, and accumulation of NCD risk caused by habitual lifetime behaviour as well as genetic factors. There is great individual variation in the rate of decline of functional ability.

However, regardless of this individual variation, there appears to be an ultimate life span limit for all humans at around 115–120 years (based on the most recent statistical estimations; Hekimi and Guarente 2003; Dong et al. 2016). Fries's survival curves (Fries 1980) supported this conclusion, as do Japan's current survival curves (MHLW of Japan 2020a) (Figure 1.10).

Figure 1.11 shows how the leading causes of death have changed over time in Japan. A clear disease shift can be seen after World War II, when infectious diseases were rapidly brought under control due to improvements in sanitation and nutrition, and NCDs such as cancer and heart disease began their steady rise along with economic development and ageing (MHLW of Japan 2020b).

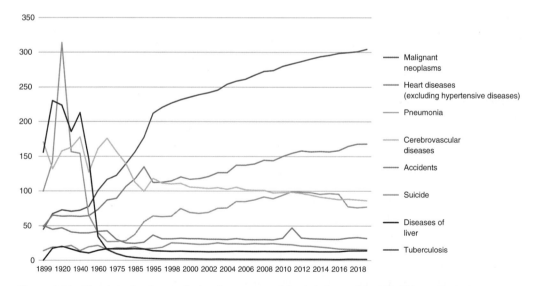

Figure 1.11 Trends in death rates for leading causes of death in Japan (per 100 000 population). *Source:* Vital Statistics, Statistics and Information Department, Minister's Secretariat, Ministry of Health, Labour and Welfare of Japan. Note: the figures for 2020 are approximate.

The main causes of death (disease structure) have changed throughout history. People used to die of starvation, accidents, violence and war. As the world became more peaceful and industrialization proceeded, infectious diseases became the leading cause of death. Scientific and medical advancements, along with public health measures, succeeded in reducing the prevalence of infectious diseases, resulting in the current situation, where NCDs have become the top killer (WHO 2020).

However, as the COVID-19 pandemic illustrated, a new infectious disease can cause a new global pandemic at any time. Low-income countries must deal with a triple burden of continuing high infectious disease rates, increasing NCDs and containment of newly emerging infectious diseases.

In the 20th century, the leading causes of death were starkly different between developed (infectious diseases) and developing (NCDs) countries. That situation, however, is rapidly changing and NCDs are already dominating as the leading causes of death in developing countries as well (WHO 2020). For this reason, preventing the occurrence and spread of NCDs such as cardiovascular diseases, cancer and diabetes mellitus is an important health policy issue in both high-income countries and LMICs.

1.4 Ageing and decline in the functions of daily living

Apart from diseases, other causes of death include ageing and accidents. When cells and organ tissue (which are groups of cells) and organs can no longer function, humans become incapable of maintaining their bodily functions as an individual organism, resulting in death. In fact, a review of the causes of individual deaths reveals that death occurs when any of the vital organs (those needed for maintaining life), such as the heart, brain, kidney and various blood vessels, can no longer function. Moreover, the process leading to death varies depending on which disease is causing that decline in organ function. For example, in the case of cerebrovascular disease, the time from becoming unable to carry out normal activities of daily living (ADLs) until the time of death is quite long (and accompanied by gradual decline). In the case of cancer, however, ADLs may be relatively normal until there is a sudden and swift decline just before death (Lynn 2001).

Ageing, therefore, is defined as a gradually progressive decline in physical functions. Ageing at the organ level can be attributed to damage to certain types of cells which have almost no ability to divide, such as brain cells, nerve cells and myocardial cells. In other cases, ageing occurs when cells stop dividing after completing approximately 50 cycles of sub-division, a phenomenon seen in almost all organs other than the abovementioned ones (Hayflick and Moorehead 1961). Either way, all organs age as one gets older, and organ ageing manifests itself in the form of reduced function. This directly causes age-related decline in muscle strength, nerve conduction velocity, lung capacity and resistance to disease, and this decline cannot be avoided in humans. For example, when evaluating age-related change in grip strength in the Japanese population, a decrease of about 12 kg in men and about 6 kg in women was observed between late-middle age and old age (MHLW of Japan 2021c) (Figure 1.12). Moreover, the percentage of essential organ function remaining at age 80 (at age 30 it is 100%) is 80% for nerve conduction velocity, less than 60% for lung capacity and renal plasma flow, and approximately 40% for maximal voluntary ventilation (Kagawa 1996). Despite this decline in organ function due to ageing, organs function together as a system, in a complementary and compensatory manner, in order to adequately support everyday

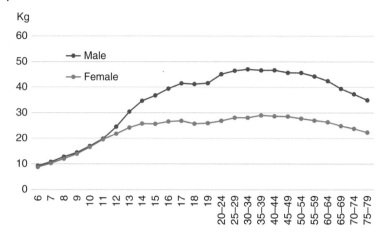

Figure 1.12 Average grip strength of Japanese by age. *Source:* Data from Ministry of Health, Labour and Welfare, 2021, Portal site of Statistics of Japan.

living functions. However, as ageing progresses, a combination of physical and psychological symptoms and conditions, collectively referred to as geriatric syndrome, are commonly observed in older adults (Sasaki 2008).

1.5   Average life expectancy (LE) and healthy life expectancy (HLE)

1.5.1   The gap between LE and HLE

The world's average life expectancy as of 2012 was 68 years in men and 73 years in women, with a mean of 70 years for both sexes combined. In contrast to the average life expectancy of 60 years in men and 63 years in women in low-income countries, the life expectancy in high-income countries reaches 76 years and 82 years, respectively. The average life expectancy of both sexes combined is 62 years in low-income countries, 66 years in low-middle-income countries, 74 years in high-middle-income countries and 79 years in high-income countries, indicating that life expectancy extends with economic development. By contrast, the global average HLE is 63.3 years, and the average HLE by economic status is 53, 57, 66 and 70 years, respectively (WHO 2014, 2020c) (Figures 1.13 and 1.14). There is an approximately 8-year difference between life expectancy and HLE, and this gap is consistent regardless of a country's economic status.

In Japan, HLE is defined as extending through the period of life in which there are no restrictions on the ADLs. Under Japan's Long-term Care Insurance System, this definition excludes those at Care Level 1 (requiring partial care due to a decline in the ability to perform basic self-care tasks and other ADLs) or above. Japan's HLE in 2019 was 72.7 years in men and 75.4 years in women, which is 8.7 years and 12.1 years lower, respectively, than the average life expectancy. Of the 36.21 million people aged 65 years and over, 4.71 million (13.0%) are at Care Level 1 or above (Cabinet Office, Japan 2022).

The diseases that most commonly lead to a condition requiring long-term care are presented in Figure 1.15. Dementia is responsible 17.6% of the time, cerebrovascular diseases 16.1% of the time, fractures/falls 12.5% and articular disease 10.8% (Figure 1.13).

1.5.2 Prolonging HLE

Life expectancy increases in tandem with economic development. And to be sure, increasing life expectancy is the primary goal of public health policy. As seen in Figures 1.14 and 1.15 (WHO 2014, 2020a), from a population standpoint, increased life expectancy *always* means increased HLE. However, the gap between HLE and actual life expectancy remains remarkably constant at around 9 years, no matter the economic status of the country or the region of the world it is in. One of the goals of global public health, therefore, should be to ensure the provision of health and well-being during these years. This can be accomplished with a two-pronged approach that combines

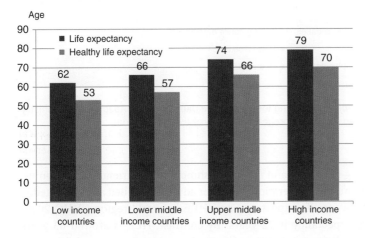

Figure 1.13 Life expectancy and healthy life expectancy by economic status. *Source:* World Health Organization 2014 / with permission of World Health Organization.

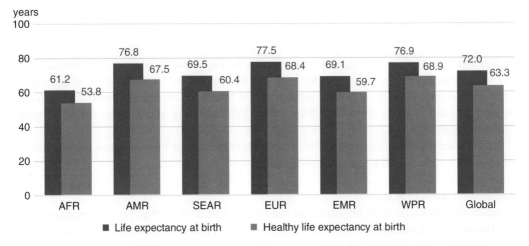

AFR: African Region, AMR: Region of the Americas, SEAR: South-East Asia Region, EUR: European Region, EMR: Eastern Mediterranean Region, WPR: Western Pacific Region

Figure 1.14 The gap between life expectancy and healthy life expectancy. *Source:* World Health Organization 2020c / with permission of World Health Organization.

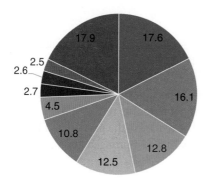

Dementia
Cerebrovascular diseases
Ageing senile detrioration
Bone fracture/falling
Articular disease
Heart diseases
Respiratory diseases
Malignant neoplasms
Diabetes
Others

Figure 1.15 Causes leading to a condition requiring long-term care (Japan). *Source:* Adapted from Ministry of Health, Labour and Welfare of Japan, 2019, Comprehensive survey of living conditions.

the provision of high-quality, long-term care and the establishment of age-friendly communities where all people live together in mutual cooperation and older adults are valued and respected.

Figure 1.14 shows the gap between life expectancy and HLE by world region (WHO 2020). The current world average life expectancy is 72 years. By contrast, HLE is around 63 years. There is an approximately 9-year difference between life expectancy and HLE, and this gap is fairly consistent regardless of a country's economic status and healthcare system. Therefore, we need to take collective action to narrow this gap so that we can have not just a 'longer life' but a 'longer, better life'.

1.5.3   Measuring HLE around the world

HLE is a generic term that is generally used for the average time people can be expected to live in a given state of health. There are three ways to measure HLE: 'average period of time spent without limitation in daily activities', 'average period of time individuals consider themselves to be healthy' and 'average period of time spent independently engaging in daily activities' (Hashimoto 2014).

However, various countries use their own methods of measuring this construct, so care must be taken when comparing HLE data among countries.

Japanese indicators of HLE

In Japan, the Health Japan 21 project established three indicators of HLE. The underlying concept and the method of measurement of these three indicators are described here. All three methods are calculated using Sullivan's method.

The first, 'average period of time spent without limitations on daily activities', defines health as the absence of limitations on daily activities. It is measured by asking the following question: 'Do you currently have any restrictions on your daily life due to health problems?' A negative answer indicates a healthy state, and an affirmative answer indicates an unhealthy state. There is also a supplementary question asking about the presence or absence of restrictions for specific activities, although this is not used for calculating the indicator. The data generated from this supplementary question can be used to implement evidence-based health promotion activities that are more effectively targeted, thus contributing to the prevention of serious diseases and the prevention of dependency on long-term care.

The second indicator is 'the average period of time individuals consider themselves to be healthy'. Here, the state of health is defined as being aware that you are healthy. It is measured by asking, 'How is your current health?' and providing five answer choices: 'very good', 'good' and 'normal' are taken as an indication that the respondent is healthy, while 'not very good' and 'not good' indicate an unhealthy state.

The third indicator is 'average period of time spent independently engaged in daily activities'. This indicator defines a healthy state as a certain degree of independence in daily living activities. Those determined to be at levels 2–5 in terms of the degree of long-term care required are considered to be unhealthy and thereby eligible for long-term care insurance, while all others are considered to be in a state of health (independence). This indicator can also be called 'average daily self-reliance period'.

European indicators of HLE

Three methods of measuring HLE have been developed under the European Community Health Indicators Monitoring system. The underlying concept and the method of measurement of these three indicators are described here. All three methods are calculated using Sullivan's method.

The first, 'life expectancy without activity limitation', defines health as the absence of long-term limitations on daily activities. It is measured by asking the following question: 'For the past 6 months or longer, have your everyday activities been continually limited by a health problem?' (Answer choices are 'yes, strongly limited', 'yes, limited' and 'no, not limited').

The second, 'life expectancy in good perceived health', defines health as good perceived health. It is measured by asking the following question: 'How is your health in general?' (Answer choices are 'very good', 'good', 'fair', 'bad', and 'very bad').

The third, 'life expectancy without chronic morbidity', defines health as the absence of self-reported chronic disease. It is measured by asking the following question: 'Do you have any longstanding illnesses or health problems?' (Answer choices are 'yes' or 'no'). Longstanding problems are defined as those which have lasted or are expected to last for 6 months or longer.

US indicators of HLE

In the US, the Healthy People 2020 goals established three methods of measuring HLE. The underlying concept and the method of measurement of these three indicators are described here. All three methods are calculated using Sullivan's method.

The first, 'expected years of life free from activity limitations', defines health as the absence of long-term restrictions on a person's everyday activities. It is measured by asking people to indicate whether they have trouble performing the following activities:

1) Activities of daily living (bathing/showering, dressing, eating, getting in and out of bed, walking, using the toilet).
2) Instrumental activities of daily living (using the telephone, doing light housework, doing heavy housework, preparing meals, shopping for personal items, managing money).
3) Play, school, or work.

4) Remembering.

5) Any other activity that they cannot do because of limitations caused by physical, mental, or emotional problems.

The second, 'expected years of life in good health', defines health as 'good perceived health'. Answer choices are 'excellent', 'very good', 'good', 'fair' or 'poor'.

The third, 'expected years of life free of certain chronic diseases', defines health as the absence of chronic disease. It is measured by asking people whether they have been diagnosed with the following six diseases: cardiovascular disease, arthritis, diabetes, asthma, cancer, and chronic obstructive pulmonary disease.

WHO indicators of HLE

The WHO estimates the effect of various diseases and health statuses on a person's health, and uses this information to calculate an individual's health-adjusted life expectancy (HALE), which can be used for international comparisons or for other public health purposes. However, the method of calculation is very complex, and ethical concerns have been raised about this purely quantitative, black-and-white determination of the effect of specific diseases on individuals' health. It has also been difficult to obtain consensus on the details of the weighting system employed with this method.

HALE is an index of HLE calculated by the WHO. Other indicators of HLE, such as those used in Japan, the US and Europe, view health as a binary proposition (health vs absence of health), but HALE views health as the ideal condition, which is chipped away at by the various injuries, illnesses, disabilities, and so on that an individual experiences during their lifetime. This allows researchers to determine the percentage of healthy or unhealthy people within a given population and to compare the health of different populations with each other. It also allows for a more fine-grained assessment of 'unhealthiness' than the indicators previously described. Most recently, the Global Burden of Disease (GBD) (2015) study applied these weighted indices to a survey of more than 60 000 people and prior studies of 315 types of poor health status, disease and disability to calculate the HALE of 195 countries and regions (Hashimoto 2014).

1.6 Strategy for healthy ageing: how to achieve healthy ageing?

In 2020, the WHO published its 'Decade of Healthy Ageing (2020–2030)' plan, which called for a decade of coordinated, catalytic and sustained cooperation (WHO 2019a,b, 2020a). Older people themselves are at the centre of this plan, which brings together governments, the citizenry, international organisations, experts, the media and the private sector to improve the lives of older people, their families and their communities. It is the second action plan of the WHO Global Strategy on Ageing and Health, which builds on the UN Madrid International Plan of Action on Ageing and aligns with the timing of the UN Sustainable Development Agenda 2030 and the Sustainable Development Goals. Oral health is given a prominent role in the report: 'Oral health is a key indicator of overall health in older age. Better integration of oral health care into general health care systems is required.'

Indicators of progress in healthy ageing, including both process and outcome indicators, are presented in Table 1.1. These indicators do not include disease-specific indicators or specific risk factors as reported by WHO. Many of the Sustainable Development Goals indicators endorsed by the member states differ by age. Having more indicators that differ by age would provide valuable information about which areas of action are most needed during this decade (WHO 2020b).

The number of countries in each global region that have reported achievement of each progress indicator as of 2020 are shown in Figure 1.16. These data indicate that provision of assistive

Table 1.1 Indicators of progress in healthy ageing, by process and outcome.

Indicator	Process	Outcome
Global strategy on ageing and health		
Countries appoint a national focal point on ageing and health in the ministry of health.	×	
Countries report a national plan on ageing and health.	×	
Countries report a national multi-stakeholder forum.	×	
Countries report national legislation and enforcement strategies against discrimination by age.	×	
Countries report national regulations or legislation on access to assistive devices.	×	
Countries report a national programme to foster age-friendly environments.	×	
Countries report a national policy to support comprehensive assessments of older people.	×	
Countries report a national policy on long-term care.	×	
Countries report the availability of national data on the health status and needs of older people.	×	
Countries report the availability of longitudinal data on the health status and needs of older people.	×	
Each country reports healthy ageing (functional ability, environment and intrinsic capacity) by age and sex.		×
WHO General Programme of Work or Core 100 indicators		
Each country reports healthy life expectancy at birth and at older ages (60, 65, 70 years, etc.).		×

Source: World Health Organization, 3 August 2020/ with permission of World Health Organization.

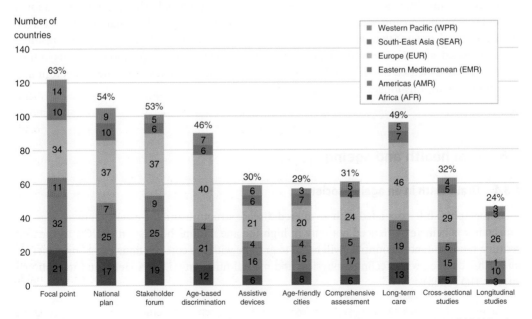

Figure 1.16 Number of countries responding 'yes' to each indicator by region and percentage of 194 Member States, 2020. *Source:* World Health Organization 2021 / with permission of World Health Organization.

devices, creation of age-friendly urban environments, and implementation of comprehensive screening programmes and research funding are urgently needed in order to make progress toward achieving healthy ageing societies (WHO 2020a).

1.7 Ageing society and social security

Improvements in pensions, medical insurance and long-term care insurance programmes are essential for older adults to live a secure life. In Japan, which as of 2024 has the longest average life span in the world, universal national health insurance and pension systems were started in 1961 and have been maintained up to the present time. Japan's insurance and pension systems are funded by both insurance fees and tax revenues, and they also function to redistribute income among age groups. These systems have played an outsized role in improving the health of the Japanese people and extending their life expectancy. Nevertheless, the combined effects of rapid population ageing and a falling birth rate place an enormous financial burden on the country (Reich et al. 2011).

Underlying generational dynamics are key to understanding population ageing in Japan. With the so-called 'baby boomers' (born in 1947–1949) turning 65 years old in 2012, the number of people aged 65 years and over reached 30.74 million, topping the 30 million mark for the first time ever. As a result, Japan has become a super-ageing society, with the percentage of the population aged 65 years and over reaching 24.1%. People aged 65–74 years account for 12.2% of the population, and those aged 75 years and over account for 11.9% of the population. In 2035, when the baby boomers reach the current average life expectancy, the percentage of the population aged 65 years and over will be 33.4% (MHLW of Japan 2013).

Meanwhile, the total expense of social security benefits in Japan reached 107.5 trillion yen in fiscal year 2011. This can be broken down to 53.06 trillion yen for pensions (49.4%), 34.06 trillion yen for medical care (31.7%) and 7.89 trillion yen for long-term care (7.3%). These numbers have increased continually since 1950, when the government started publishing this data (National Institute of Population and Social Security Research 2014. The irony of the situation is that it is the success of these systems that has resulted in the increasing expenses. These systems have resulted in an increased survival rate accompanied by the rapid ageing of the population, and this in turn has drastically increased the financial burden of maintaining the systems and thereby continuing to improve the healthy longevity of the population.

1.8 Oral health and ageing

1.8.1 Oral health in an ageing society

A demographic shift associated with an altered disease structure and the extension in average life expectancy is being experienced not only in high-income nations but also in LMICs. In the 21st century, more and more countries will begin to grapple with the core dilemma of ageing societies: longer life coupled with declining physical and mental function (UNFPA HelpAge International 2012; WHO 2020b).

Oral function is essential for the maintenance of QOL, particularly the functions of eating and communication (Fukai et al. 2022). For this reason, the ultimate goal should be the establishment of a global health system in which all people can receive dental care and oral health services throughout their entire lifetime, irrespective of the region or country in which they live. Moreover, scientific evidence has been accumulating that shows the effectiveness of dental care and oral health in preventing disease in organs other than the oral cavity and in maintaining general health. It is therefore generally accepted that dental care and oral health can and must play an essential role in solving the multifaceted health problems that our ageing society is facing, and that giving due consideration to dental care and oral health in each country's health policies will lead to better and more comprehensive solutions to our health problems (Salomon et al. 2012; GBD 2017 DALYs and HALE Collaborators 2018).

This section is an attempt to document the current status of global population ageing, not only in high-income countries but also in LMICs, and to postulate a conceptual pathway linking improved oral care to improved general health and HLE.

The analysis presented in this section is based on a broad, ongoing synthesis of research on HLE and social security systems, as well as a comprehensive review of dental/oral and general health investigations combined with statistical data provided by public institutions.

1.8.2 Oral health and HLE

An accumulation of evidence has established a strong relationship between oral and general health, and there are two general pathways whereby dental care and oral health contribute to healthy longevity: (1) health promotion activities and (2) reduction in the risk of disease. The first pathway involves promotion of healthy behaviour such as exercise, nutrition and rest. The second pathway involves reducing risk factors for NCDs and preventing the onset and worsening of diseases that lead to death or long-term care.

Figure 1.17 shows the decline in the average number of teeth with age in the Japanese population from 1957 to 2016. The curve has moved to the right over time, which means people are keeping their teeth and oral function until older ages. For example, the average female had just 20 remaining teeth at age 40 in 1957, but 60 years later, she still has 27 remaining teeth at age 40, and the number of teeth does not fall below 20 until after age 70. This means that people today have an oral health status that would have been characteristic of someone 30 years younger just 60 years ago (Fukai et al. 2011).

At the same time, an analysis of the slopes of these curves using an optimal regression equation reveals that the number of years it takes go from 25 to five teeth or 20 to 10 teeth has not changed much over the past 60 years. Therefore, it is important to avoid the slippery slope of tooth loss through early life course intervention for tooth loss prevention.

Figure 1.18 shows the relationship between number of teeth and longevity from in the Japanese population from 1957 to 2005 using national data. It shows that people lose approximately half of their teeth between the ages of 65 and 74. Of course, a close relationship between life expectancy and number of teeth does not mean that number of teeth is the only factor in increasing life expectancy. Rather, increased life expectancy year-by-year suggests increased general health and increased quality of healthcare, of which dental health is an integral part (Fukai 2010).

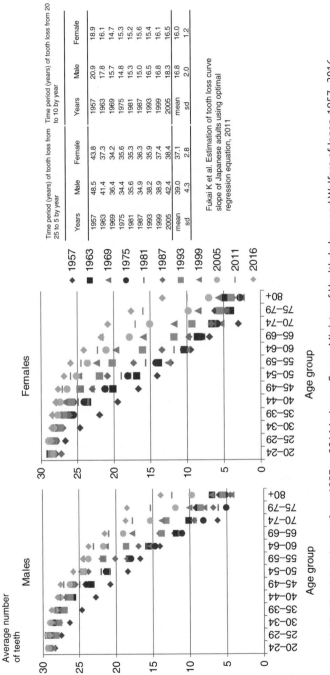

Figure 1.17 Tooth loss by age from 1957 to 2016 in Japan. *Source:* Ministry of Health, Labour and Welfare of Japan, 1957–2016.

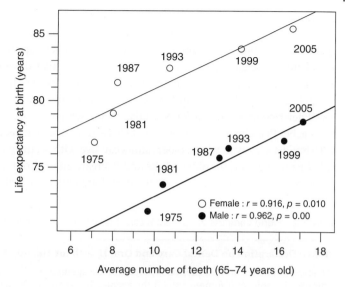

Figure 1.18 Oral health and longevity: relationship between tooth number and life expectancy during the past 30 years (1975–2005). *Source:* Fukai. K. et al. 2010 / John Wiley & Sons.

1.9 Challenges of general health and oral health in an ageing society

Global population ageing is an unstoppable phenomenon; the most important challenge facing us now is how to prolong the healthy period of human life.

The survival curve of the Japanese population by gender and age was presented in this chapter. The survival rate at age 80 years is approximately 80% for women and 60% for men. This means that the number of deaths actually peaks at age 85 years in men and 91 years in women. The death rate increases linearly (log plot) with age from about 30 to 90 years old. This is known as the Gompertz law (1825), which states that 'the probability of death exponentially increases with age'. There is a two-fold increase in the probability of death every 8 years from age 30, and an 80-year-old is 30 times more likely to die than a 40-year-old. Gompertz also defined ageing as 'increased susceptibility to death'. Ageing makes humans more susceptible to death and disease.

The world's oldest living person on record was a French woman called Calmant, who died at the age of 122 in 1997, and the life span of human beings is considered to be limited to around 120 years (Dong et al. 2016). The drop-off portion of the survival curve becomes markedly steeper in ageing societies, as a higher and higher percentage of the population lives past the average life span (Hekimi et al. 2003). This steep drop-off is a clear indicator that a society is achieving the goal of bringing the average life expectancy closer to the biological limit of the human life span (and increasing HLE as well). The key to achieving this goal is to take preventive measures against the leading causes of death while implementing health promotion activities aimed at preventing senescence. In order to further enhance population health, it is important to implement policies that effectively reduce risk factors such as hyperglycaemia, lack of exercise, drinking, overweight/obese status, high intake of salt, high blood pressure and smoking (Ikeda et al. 2011). It is also important to identify which diseases most often lead to the need for long-term care and to prevent such diseases.

In order to keep social security costs at manageable levels, a system that effectively and efficiently reduces preventable diseases is needed. The factors that damage health are genetic and those related to lifestyle, social security/health system and social environment. Among these, genetic factors contribute to about 25–30% of all deaths (Schroeder 2007; Christensen et al. 2009). However, when evaluating overall disease risk, lifestyle and social environments turn out to be more important than genetic background. For example, in a well-known follow-up study of Japanese Americans on the prevalence of ischaemic heart disease and cerebrovascular disease, the Japanese Americans (first-generation immigrants) were reported to have a higher risk of ischaemic heart disease and a lower risk of cerebrovascular disease than Japanese living in Japan (Takeya et al. 1984). Because behaviour and social determinants account for NCD risk to a much greater extent than genetic factors, preventive approaches that aim to reduce the risk of NCDs should be pursued.

To build a society in which older adults can live with security and dignity, it is important to provide income support for older adults and to create an environment where they are encouraged to participate in social activities (FDI 2018; Foreman et al. 2018; GBD 2017 Causes of Death

Table 1.2   World Congress 2015: dental care and oral health for healthy longevity in an ageing society.

Tokyo Declaration on Dental Care and Oral Health for Healthy Longevity

In many countries around the world, societies are ageing rapidly as medical advances and an improved living environment extend the average life span. At the same time, this has generated a marked discrepancy between actual life expectancy and the expectancy of healthy life, resulting in a complex situation in which the number of people needing nursing care has increased. Inevitably societies face, as a consequence, the task of preventing the decline in the quality of life of people who need nursing care.

The challenge is to develop the role of dental care and oral health in creating societies with healthy longevity. Dental care should respond to the problem of increased non-communicable diseases as living environments change and should expand its support for people who need nursing care and preventing premature death. Dental associations and other health professionals around the world are encouraged to facilitate and enhance coordination of activities to increase global awareness of and contribute to the implementation of WHO's Global Action Plan for the Prevention and Control of Noncommunicable Diseases 2013–2030.

Life-long oral health is a fundamental human right, underpinned by an 'oral-health-in-all-policies' approach.

The World Congress 2015 adopted the Tokyo Declaration on Dental Care and Oral Health for Healthy Longevity, calling for:

1) A concerted effort to accumulate scientific evidence of the contribution of dental care and oral health to longer healthy life expectancy and to formulate health policies based on such evidence.

2) Further investigation into the status of national dental health care policies and regional health activities supported by such evidence, with the sharing of results and related information among countries across the world.

3) Recognition that maintenance of oral and dental health throughout life is a fundamental factor for improving quality of life, helping to protect against non-communicable diseases and contributing towards preventing the aggravation of such diseases – it can also contribute to longer healthy life expectancy.

4) Community dental care providers and institutions to play a fundamental role in ensuring that, in ageing societies, appropriate dental care is provided at all stages of life and that concerted efforts to put oral health into practice are made at the national level.

5) An understanding that health policy should focus on how to recognize risks common to both oral diseases and non-communicable diseases in order to devise a common risk factor approach, prevent oral diseases and tooth loss, and maintain and revitalize oral function by a life-course approach.

6) An appreciation that, in order to contribute to preventing both non-communicable diseases and a decline in oral function in old age, dental and other health professionals must create an environment that enables and encourages multi-professional collaborative practice.

Source: Adapted from Kakuhiro Fukai 2015.

Collaborators 2018; WHO 2018). One of the most important goals for both high-income countries and LMICs should be to create a system in which older adults can receive high-quality healthcare services based on collaboration between the medical and dental fields.

Oral health throughout the life course is now seen throughout the world as a fundamental and essential component of socioeconomic development. The starting point for this discussion was the 2015 World Congress on Oral Health and Ageing, which was held jointly by the Japan Dental Association (JDA) and the WHO in Tokyo, Japan. At this congress, the 'Tokyo Declaration on Dental Care and Oral Health for Healthy Longevity' (Table 1.2) was issued, establishing a clear link between both NCD prevention and frailty, on the one hand, and oral health prevention on the other (JDA 2015). It also stressed the importance of multisectorial efforts in this area. In order to make concrete progress on the goals set out in this declaration, the World Dental Federation's (FDI) Oral Health for an Ageing Population (OHAP) task team was formed (https://www.fdiworlddental.org/oral-health-ageing-population). During the first stage of OHAP, the task team set out to raise awareness of the importance of oral health in confronting the challenges of the ageing society phenomenon, providing practical recommendations (including a roadmap) to that end. During the second stage of the OHAP, the team set out to develop concrete solutions to these challenges (GBD 2017 DALYs and HALE Collaborators 2018).

1.10 Conclusion

In order to attain a healthy ageing society, the currently available scientific evidence showing the contribution of dental care and oral health to general health must be recognized and applied in policy and practice, and further research in this area must be promoted. There is an urgent need to verify the effects of dental care and oral health on various factors impairing general health and to implement sound new policies based on the accumulated evidence.

In order to realize healthy longevity in our society, the following four objectives should be established: (1) to increase life expectancy and prevent early death; (2) to prevent people from becoming dependent on long-term care; (3) to slow the decline in daily living functions that accompanies ageing; and (4) to promote healthy behaviour from the early years of adulthood based on the life course approach.

References

Beard, J.R. (2016). The world report on ageing and health: a policy framework for healthy ageing, *Lancet*, 387(10033), 2145–2154.

Cabinet Office (2022). Annual report on the ageing society. Tokyo: Cabinet Office.

Christensen, K., Doblhammer, G., Rau, R., & Vaupel, JW. (2009). Ageing populations, the challenges ahead. *Lancet*, 374, 1196–1208.

Dong, X., Milholland, B., & Vijg, J. (2016) Evidence for a limit to human lifespan. *Nature*, 538, 257–259.

FDI World Dental Federation (2018). Oral health for an ageing population: Roadmap for healthy ageing, Geneva, FDI. https://www.fdiworlddental.org/roadmap-healthy-ageing (accessed 24 June 2024).

Foreman, K.J., Marquez, N., Dolgert, A. et al. (2018). Forecasting life expectancy, years of life lost, and all-cause and cause-specific mortality for 250 causes of death: reference and alternative scenarios for 2016-40 for 195 countries and territories. *Lancet*, 392(10159), 2052–2090. https://www.thelancet.com/action/showPdf?pii=S0140-6736%2818%2931694-5 (accessed 17 October 2023).

Fries, J.F. (1980). Aging, natural death, and the compression of morbidity. *N Engl J Med*, 303, 130–135.

Fukai, K. (2015). Oral health in an aging society, Japan Dental Association (Fukai K. editor-in chief) The current evidence of dental care and oral health for achieving healthy longevity in an aging society. Japan Dental Association,16–22.

Fukai, K. et al. (2011). Estimation of tooth loss curve slope of Japanese adults using optimal regression equation (in Japanese). Research report on the appropriate number of dentists based on the forecasted demand for dental diseases and the demand of patients and others. MHLW Grants System, pp. 141–148. https://mhlw-grants.niph.go.jp/system/files/2010/104011/201031014A/201031014A0008.pdf (accessed 24 June 2024).

Fukai, K. (2013) Future directions for research on the contributions of dental and oral health to a healthy aging society. *Health Sci Health Care*, 13(2), 39–42. https://www.fihs.org/volume13_2/editorial1.pdf (accessed 24 June 2024).

Fukai, K., Dartevelle, S., Jones, J. (2022 August) Oral health for healthy ageing: a people-centred and function-focused approach. *Int Dent J*, 72(4S), S2–S4.

Fukai, K., Takiguchi, T., Sasaki, H. (2010). Dental health and longevity. *Geriatr Gerontol Int*, 10 275–10 276.

Global Burden of Disease (GBD) 2015 Disease and Injury Incidence and Prevalence Collaborators. (2015). Global, regional, and national life expectancy, all-cause mortality, and cause-specific mortality for 249 causes of death, 1980-2015: a systematic analysis for the Global Burden of Disease Study 2015. *Lancet*, 388(10053), 1459–1544.

Global Burden of Disease (GBD) 2017 Causes of Death Collaborators. (2018). Global, regional, and national age-sex-specific mortality for 282 causes of death in 195 countries and territories, 1980-2017: a systematic analysis for the Global Burden of Disease Study 2017. *Lancet*, 392(10159), 1736–1788. https://www.thelancet.com/action/showPdf?pii=S0140-6736%2818%2932203-7 (accessed 8 July 2024).

Global Burden of Disease (GBD) 2017 DALYs and HALE Collaborators. (2018). Global, regional, and national disability-adjusted life-years (DALYs) for 359 diseases and injuries and healthy life expectancy (HALE) for 195 countries and territories, 1990–2017: a systematic analysis for the Global Burden of Disease Study 2017. *Lancet*, 392(10159), 1859–1922.

Hashimoto, S. (2015 March). Research on the current status and analytical assessment of healthy life expectancy in Japan and overseas. (in Japanese). MHLW Grants System. http://toukei.umin.jp/kenkoujyumyou/houkoku/H26_toku.pdf (accessed 13 May 2024).

Hayflick, L., Moorhead, P.S. (1961). The serial cultivation of human diploid cell strains. *Exp Cell Res*, 25, 585–621.

Hekimi, S., Guarente, L. (2003). Genetics and the specificity of the aging process. *Science*, 299(5611), 1351–1354.

Ikeda, N., Saito, E., Kondo, N. et al. (2011). What has made the population of Japan healthy? *Lancet*, 378(9796), 1094–105.

Japan Dental Association (JDA) (2015). The current evidence of dental care and oral health for achieving healthy longevity in an aging society 2015. Japan Dental Association.

Kagawa, Y. (1996). *Bioscience of Aging*. Tokyo: Youtosha, 24–27.

Lynn, J. (2001). Serving patients who may die soon and their families The role of hospice and other services. *J Am Med Assoc*, 285(7), 925–932.

Ministry of Health, Labour and Welfare (MHLW), Japan. (2019). *Comprehensive Survey of Living Conditions* (in Japanese). Tokyo: MHLW.

Ministry of Health, Labour and Welfare (MHLW), Japan. (2020a). *Life Table*. Tokyo: MHLW.

Ministry of Health, Labour and Welfare (MHLW), Japan, Minister's Secretariat. (2020b). *Vital Statistics*. Tokyo: MHLW, Statistics and Information Department.

Ministry of Health, Labour and Welfare (MHLW), Japan. (2021a). *Vital Statistics*. Tokyo: MHLW.

Ministry of Health, Labour and Welfare (MHLW), Japan. (2021b). *Life Table, 2021*. Tokyo: MHLW.

Ministry of Health, Labour and Welfare (MHLW), Japan. (2021c). *Portal Site of Statistics of Japan*. Tokyo: MHLW.

National Institute of Population and Social Security Research. (2014). Social Security Statistics of Japan 2012, Tokyo, National Institute of Population and Social Security Research

OECD (2019). Life expectancy and healthy life expectancy at age 65. In: *Health at a Glance 2019*: *OECD Indicators*. OECD Publishing. https://www.oecd-ilibrary.org/sites/82ca511d-en/index.html?itemId=/content/component/82ca511d-en (accessed 13 May 2024).

Reich, M.R., Ikegami, N., Shibuya, K., & Takemi, K. (2011). 50 years of pursuing a healthy society in Japan. *Lancet*, 378(9796), 1051–1053.

Salomon, J. A., Wang, H., Freeman, M. K. et al. (2012). Healthy life expectancy for 187 countries, 1990–2010: a systematic analysis for the Global Burden Disease Study 2010. *Lancet*, 380(9859), 2144–2162. https://www.thelancet.com/pdfs/journals/lancet/PIIS0140-6736(19)30041-8.pdf (accessed 13 May 2024).

Sasaki, H. (2008). Single pathogenesis of geriatric syndrome. *Geriatr Gerontol Int*, 8(1), 1–4.

Schroeder, S.A. (2007). We can do better - Improving the health of the American people. *N Engl J Med*, 357(12), 1221–1228.

Takeya, Y. et al. (1984). Epidemiologic studies of coronary heart disease and stroke in Japanese men living in Japan, Hawaii and California: incidence of stroke in Japan and Hawaii. *Stroke*, 15(1), 15–23.

United Nations Population Fund (UNFPA) and HelpAge International. (2012). *Ageing in the Twenty-First Century: A Celebration and A Challenge Executive Summary*. New York: UNFPA. https://www.unfpa.org/sites/default/files/pub-pdf/Ageing%20report.pdf (accessed 13 May 2024).

United Nations. (2019). *World Population Prospects*. New York: UN.

United Nations. (2022). *World Population Prospects*, New York: UN. https://population.un.org/wpp/ (accessed 13 May 2024).

World Health Organization. (2011). *Global Status Report on Noncommunicable Diseases 2010*. WHO Library. Geneva: WHO.

World Health Organization. (2014). *World Health Statistics 2014*. WHO Library. Geneva: WHO.

World Health Organization. (2018). *Health Statistics and Information Systems Metrics: Disability-adjusted Life Year (DALY) Quantifying the Burden of Disease from Mortality and Morbidity*. Geneva: WHO.

World Health Organization. (2019a). Risk reduction of cognitive decline and dementia. *WHO Guideline*. Geneva: WHO.

World Health Organization. (2019b). WHO Clinical Consortium on Healthy Ageing 2019: report of Consortium meeting held 21-22 November 2019 in Geneva, Switzerland. https://www.who.int/publications/i/item/9789240009752 (accessed 13 May 2024).

World Health Organization. (2020a). *Decade of Healthy Ageing Baseline Report*. Geneva: WHO. https://www.who.int/publications/i/item/9789240017900 (accessed 13 May 2024).

World Health Organization. (2020b). *Decade of Healthy Ageing 2020–2030: Plan Of Action*. Geneva: WHO. https://www.who.int/publications/m/item/decade-of-healthy-ageing-plan-of-action

World Health Organization. (2020c). *World Health Statics 2020*. Geneva: WHO.

World Health Organization. (2020d). The top 10 causes of death. *WHO Fact Sheet*. Geneva: WHO. https://www.who.int/en/news-room/fact-sheets/detail/the-top-10-causes-of-death

2

Achieving oral health among older adults: Community and clinical approaches

Oral Health for an Ageing Population: Evidence, Policy, Practice and Evaluation, First Edition. Kakuhiro Fukai.
© 2025 John Wiley & Sons Ltd. Published 2025 by John Wiley & Sons Ltd.

2.1 Introduction

Oral diseases have a higher prevalence than systemic diseases (Kassebaum et al. 2017; GBD 2017 Oral Disorders Collaborators 2020; WHO 2022) (Figures 2.1 and 2.2). The oral health of older people is particularly affected by tooth loss, which results from the accumulation of dental caries and worsening periodontal disease throughout one's life. Even when not accompanied by tooth loss, dental caries and periodontal disease themselves are also significant health risks that negatively affect the quality of life of older people (Naito 2015). In addition, age-related decline in the muscle strength of the tongue, orbicularis oculus, and the masticatory and swallowing muscles, together with reduced saliva, leads to a gradual decline in oral function (Fukai et al. 2022). Prevention of such oral functional decline is important in its own right, and it is also important for frailty prevention, as frailty is associated with undernutrition in the elderly.

Assessment of oral health status in older people requires community-wide screening in addition to full dental examinations at dental clinics. If examinations at dental clinics are the only approach utilized, it is difficult to catch the early stages of reduced oral function in healthy people and take appropriate community and individual measures.

This chapter, therefore, focuses on the importance of cooperation between local communities and dental institutions within the larger national healthcare system, which itself must be built around a stable medical insurance system and accompanying long-term care insurance system.

In addition, cognitive function decline has become a major health challenge for ageing societies, so it is essential to consider how dental treatment and dental health guidance can be adapted specifically for people with dementia (Livingston et al. 2017). This chapter therefore describes how dental treatment can be integrated into national dementia policies, with a particular focus on the emerging role of dental care in preventing cognitive decline.

2.2 Oral health in older adults

The increasing percentage of older adults in the global population will have implications for nearly all sectors of society, including health and oral health in particular. An important implication of the United Nations 2030 Agenda for Sustainable Development is that, as populations

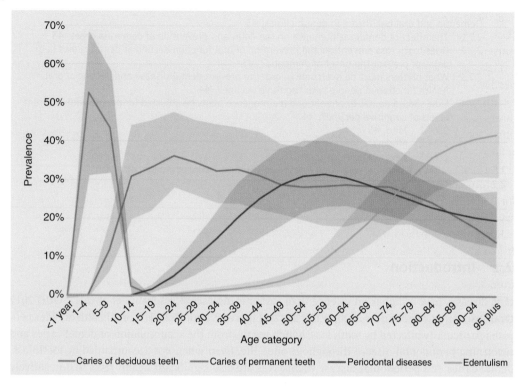

Figure 2.1 Prevalence rates of four major oral diseases over the life course. *Source:* World Health Organization (2022)/with permission of World Health Organization.

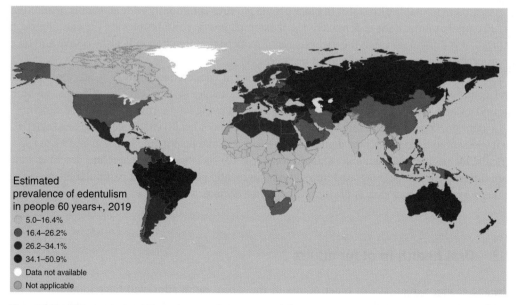

Figure 2.2 Estimated prevalence of edentulism. *Source:* World Health Organization (2022)/with permission of World Health Organization.

age, the goal of ensuring healthy lives and well-being at all ages becomes more urgent than ever (UN 2015). If oral healthcare systems are to contribute to reaching this ambitious goal, they must adapt accordingly.

The emergence of a 'society of longevity' is the result of human progress. On the other hand, the decline of vital functions and health with age is a biological process that cannot be halted. Oral health is no different. Older adults, therefore, often have complicated clinical conditions. Chronic diseases such as diabetes and respiratory diseases, polypharmacy, frailty and dependence on care often accompany physiological ageing (WHO 2015). Impaired vision, lower tactile thresholds, reduced dexterity, cognitive impairment and dementia often complicate daily oral hygiene routines (Fukai et al. 2019).

According to the Global Burden of Disease (GBD) study, oral disease in older adults accounted for 3.5 million disability-adjusted life years (DALYs), primarily due to edentulism, followed by severe periodontitis and untreated caries (Kassebaum et al. 2014a, 2015).

Edentulism impairs chewing ability and often leads to a change in diet and limited food choices. It can also affect social interactions and, more generally, quality of life. Edentulism drastically increases with age, and its prevalence strongly varies according to geographic location, ranging from 30% of those over 65 in certain regions of Latin America to only 9% in East Asia (Kassebaum et al. 2017). The prevalence of periodontal disease also gradually increases with age, and there are clear geographic differences in prevalence here as well, ranging from 51% of older adults in east Sub-Saharan Africa to 10% in Oceania (Kassebaum et al. 2015). Untreated caries also increase with age, peaking at 70 years as the risk of root caries suddenly increases (Kassebaum et al. 2014b).

2.3   Frailty and level of dependency in older adults

In 2001, Fried et al. (2001) proposed the 'frailty cycle', a vicious circle model involving decreasing muscle strength and mass (sarcopenia), fatigue and decreasing energy consumption. The model demonstrates that nutritional factors such as loss of appetite, weight loss and low nutrition are accelerators of frailty (Figure 2.3).

Frailty can be defined as a 'state of increased vulnerability to stressors due to age related decline in physiological reserve across neuromuscular, metabolic and immune systems' (Pretty et al. 2014).

The levels of dependency described in Table 2.1 are based on the Lucerne Care Pathway, which in turn is derived from the Seattle Care Pathway for maintaining oral health in older patients (Fukai et al. 2018). Recommended interventions may vary depending on the older adult's pre-assessed level of dependency for dental care teams.

Frailty and vulnerability need to be assessed at various levels: government, policy, population and individual. Figure 2.4 can be used to implement a life-course approach to oral health and to implement service delivery strategies which avoid under- and overtreatment.

2.4   Deterioration of oral health function

Healthy longevity and health equity are the right goals, and they resonate with people in all walks of life and of all races and cultures. They therefore have the potential to unite humanity across our multitudinous divisions. The factors contributing to healthy longevity are numerous, complex and interrelated, requiring creative, interdisciplinary, intergenerational and global approaches.

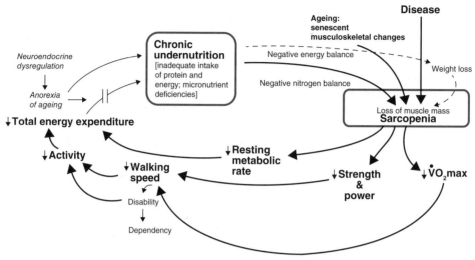

Figure 2.3 Frailty in older adults: evidence for a phenotype. *Source:* Fried L.P. et al. 2001/Oxford University Press.

Table 2.1 A definition of levels of dependency.

Level of Dependency	Definition
No dependency CSHA level 1 & 2	Robust people who exercise regularly and are the most fit group for their age.
Pre-dependency CSHA level 3	People with chronic systemic conditions that could impact oral health but, at the point of presentation, are not currently impacting oral health. A comorbidity whose symptoms are well controlled.
Low dependency CSHA level 4	People with identified chronic conditions that are affecting oral health but who currently receive or do not require help to access dental services or maintain oral health. These patients are not entirely dependent, but their disease symptoms are affecting them.
Medium dependency CSHA level 5	People with an identified chronic systemic condition that currently impacts their oral health and who receive or do not require help to access dental services or maintain oral health. This category includes patients who demand to be seen at home or who do not have transport to a dental clinic.
High dependency CSHA level 6 & 7	People who have complex medical problems preventing them from moving to receive dental care at a dental clinic. They differ from patients categorized in medium dependency because they cannot be moved and must be seen at home.

CSHA, Canadian Study of Health and Aging.
Source: FDI. Older adults chair side guide, 2019.

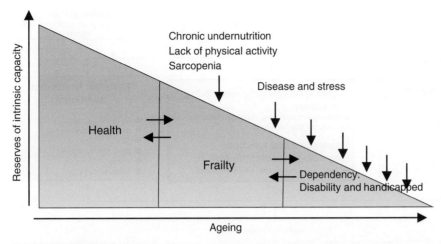

Figure 2.4 Frailty and dependency by age. *Source:* Adapted from MHLW of Japan, Guidelines for health services based on the characteristics of older people (in Japanese), 3rd ed., 2024, https://www.mhlw.go.jp/content/001240315.pdf

Prevention of oral function decline is an important part of that picture, and person-centred approaches such as community-based, muti-sectoral screening programmes are practical, effective and pose a low economic burden on society.

Ageing has become a major health challenge confronting all countries in the world at the same time, regardless of socioeconomic status. Humans have long wanted to live longer lives, but having achieved longevity, we are confronted by the reality that this celebrated achievement brings with it great challenges. Ageing causes individuals to become more susceptible to disease, leading to a decline in the essential functions of living (including both intrinsic capacity and functional ability).

According to the 2015 World Report on Ageing and Health, the goal of healthy ageing is to ensure that people can maintain the degree of functional ability required for well-being (WHO 2015). Functional ability refers to the 'health-related attributes that enable people to be and to do what they have reason to value'. Functional ability is determined by the intrinsic capacity of the individual as well as the environment of the individual and the interaction between those two factors. Intrinsic capacity is 'the composite of all the physical and mental capacities 'that an individual can draw on'. To delay functional decline and maintain health and well-being, we must provide medical care and long-term care for all, and we must also integrate those systems into a social infrastructure that encourages healthy behaviour and improves accessibility to care.

Eating, talking and smiling are essential life functions that are directly linked to oral health (Glick et al. 2016). Therefore, oral healthcare access must be viewed as a core, universal human right. This implies that communities and governments are obligated to provide a healthcare system that ensures that all people have access to the information, prevention and care needed to maintain oral health throughout their life.

Oral function is a complex system of interacting anatomical parts and movements. Most prominent are the higher-order functions needed for daily life and survival, such as eating, talking and smiling. These functions are, in turn, supported by a number of interacting lower-order physiological and functional components: teeth, saliva, lips, the tongue and other oral-facial

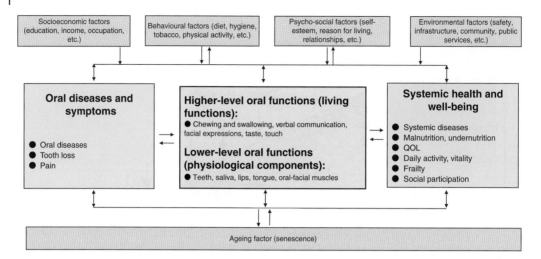

Figure 2.5 Conceptual pathway of oral function decline. *Source:* Fukai K. et al. 2002/with permission of Elsevier.

muscles. As people get older, the oral environment undergoes changes and they experience a decline in oral functions, such as motor function (lips and tongue movement) as well as chewing and swallowing function. Figure 2.5 presents a novel conceptual pathway that incorporates the complex array of factors involved in oral function decline (Fukai et al. 2022). This pathway places oral function in the centre and shows how various factors contribute to it and are affected by it. The main risk factors of oral function decline are well known: oral diseases and symptoms such as caries, periodontal disease, tooth loss and pain. However, this figure emphasizes the fact that a variety of factors related to general health and well-being also contribute in important ways to oral function decline. This figure also shows the complex reciprocal relationships between the various factors and oral function. It should further be noted that the three central elements of the pathway (oral diseases, oral functions and systemic health) are themselves constantly interacting with social and psychological factors such as economic status, behaviour and environment (including health services). Finally, the pathway indicates that all of this exists within the overarching context of the ageing process, and indeed it is an integral part of the ageing process.

The link between ageing and oral function decline, as well as the effect of oral function decline on general physical health, are based on a growing body of evidence. For example, the percentage of older Japanese people with dysphagia is reported to be 25.1% (Igarashi et al. 2019). The decline in oral function that accompanies ageing reduces the diversity of food intake, resulting in nutritional deficiency. Furthermore, a large-scale longitudinal study of Japanese older people revealed that minor oral dysfunction increases the risk of muscle loss, dependence on long-term care and death (Tanaka et al. 2018).

In order to delay the decline of oral function, the Japanese Geriatric Dental Association proposed an expanded dental screening and assessment programme that would identify even small changes in tongue and lip function, saliva production and eating functions (Minakuchi et al. 2018; Tanaka et al. 2021) (Figure 2.6). While the reliability and validity of the assessment instruments need further improvement, it is clear that there is a great need for person-centred assessment of oral function. In order to maintain oral health in the later stages of life, such assessments need to be implemented on the basis of multi-sectoral cooperation and information-sharing.

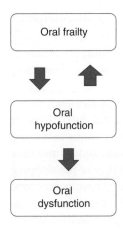

Oral frailty	JSG defines oral hypofunction based on the presentation of 7 oral signs or symptoms. The criteria for each symptom were determined based on data from previous studies, and oral hypofunction is diagnosed if the criteria for 3 or more of these signs or symptoms are met.

Poor oral hygiene	The total number of microorganisms (CFU/mL) is $10^{6.5}$ or more
Oral dryness	The measured value obtained by a recommended moisture checker is less than 27.0
Reduced occlusal force	The occlusal force is less than 200 N
Decreased tongue-lip motor function	The number of /pa/, /ta/ or /ka/ syllables produced per second is less than 6
Decreased tongue pressure	The maximum tongue pressure is less than 30 kPa
Decreased masticatory function	The glucose concentration obtained by chewing gelatin gummies is less than 100 mg/dL
Deterioration of swallowing function	The total score of EAT-10 is 3 or higher

Figure 2.6 Definition and criteria of oral hypofunction. JSG, Japanese Society of Gerodontology. *Source:* Adapted from Minakuchi S. et al., 2018.

There has already been some research on the types of interventions (for improvement of oral function) that should be implemented in tandem with such screening programmes. Types of intervention include: health education (e.g. how the oral cavity and saliva support our daily life, or how to prevent aspiration pneumonia); oral hygiene instruction; and exercises to maintain oral function (e.g. tongue and face exercises, saliva gland massage, pronunciation training and breathing exercises) (Sakayori et al. 2013; Ohara et al. 2015; Iwao et al. 2019). These interventions can be undertaken by healthcare professionals in various fields, including dental hygienists.

Evaluating the effectiveness of oral function improvement interventions for older people is an increasingly active area of research. However, systematic reviews and meta-analyses of this evidence have not yet been conducted, so establishing the effectiveness of these interventions requires further research (Dent et al. 2019).

The goals of health equity and healthy longevity resonate with people all over the world regardless of race, culture or socioeconomic status. These goals, therefore, have the potential to unite us around a common mission and vision, overcoming our divisions. There are numerous interrelated factors contributing in complex ways to healthy longevity, so we need creative, interdisciplinary, intergenerational and global approaches. Maintenance of oral function is an essential part of the solution and this requires practical, effective, low-cost, person-centred approaches such as community-based, multi-sectoral screening.

2.5 Nutrition and oral health for older adults

Many studies on frailty prevention have reported a relationship between protein intake and frailty. In the elderly, decreasing muscle mass and decline in functional ability often occur. This is partly caused by anabolic resistance, which occurs with ageing, and which in turn causes a weakening of the assimilation suppression reaction of skeletal muscle (Cruz-Jentoft et al. 2010; Chen et al. 2020).

It is important for older people to consume enough protein. It is particularly important that protein intake exceed the recommended level where nitrogen equilibrium, which is an indicator of protein metabolism, has been lost and output is greater than intake. For example, in one study, when a woman over 65 years old with frailty was put on a high-protein diet (1.23 g/kg per day), her anabolic response and nitrogen equilibrium improved, demonstrating the effectiveness of a high-protein diet. This has been confirmed in many other studies as well (Motokawa et al. 2021).

In addition, it has been shown that consuming a diverse variety of food and nutrients, rather than a limited variety, is effective in preventing frailty and sarcopenia (Kimura et al. 2103). In order to improve the diversity of food intake in daily life, it is recommended that older people be encouraged to: (1) not skip meals, (2) snack on dairy products and fruits between meals, and (3) make use of commercially prepared meals such as frozen foods. Regarding the importance of not skipping meals, Motokawa et al. (2021) reported that people who eat only twice a day have poorer food diversity and lower energy intake (by 100 kcal) than those eating three times a day. Regarding the benefit of between-meal consumption, when people experience decreased appetite and are unable to consume the recommended amount of food during meals, snacking between meals is an easy way to increase intake. When incorporating snacks, diversity of food intake can be improved by incorporating milk, other dairy products, and fruits, which tend to be insufficient in ordinary meals (Motokawa et al. 2021).

Inadequate and poor-quality diet, as well as malnutrition, are commonly associated with adverse health outcomes, including morbidity and mortality, among older people. Additionally, a large number of studies have produced a great deal of evidence on the association between nutrition and oral health. Overall, it is clear that number of teeth and dentition influence food and nutrient intake, including food diversity. For example, one study showed that the intake of vegetables and meat decreases along with the number of remaining teeth. On the other hand, intake of carbohydrates and rice increases with tooth loss (Yoshihara et al. 2005). Another study found that individuals with impaired dentition demonstrated a significantly greater degree of decline in the intake of multiple nutrients (protein, sodium, potassium, calcium, vitamin A, vitamin E and dietary fibre) than those without impaired dentition (Iwasaki et al. 2021). In yet another study, patients receiving new complete dentures were divided into two groups. The intervention group received denture care advice along with simple dietary advice from a nutritionist using a uniform pamphlet, while the control group received only denture care advice. Protein intake in the intervention group increased significantly compared with the control group (Suzuki et al. 2017).

Wakai et al. (2010) found that intake of carotene, vitamins A and C, milk and dairy products, and vegetables (including green-yellow vegetables) decreased as number of teeth decreased (p for trend < 0.05). On the other hand, mean intake of carbohydrates, rice and confectioneries increased as the number of teeth decreased (p for trend < 0.05) (Wakai et al. 2010).

Kimura et al. (2013) conducted an evaluation of chewing ability and its relationship with activities of daily living, depression, cognitive status and food intake in community-dwelling elderly people. Participants with low chewing ability consumed a lower variety of food ($p < 0.001$) and had less frequent intake of beans, vegetables, seaweed and nuts than those with high chewing ability (Kimura et al. 2013).

Iwasaki et al. (2016) found a longitudinal association of dentition status with dietary intake in Japanese adults aged 75–80 years. Individuals with impaired dentition demonstrated a significantly ($p < 0.05$) greater degree of decline in the intake of multiple nutrients (protein, sodium, potassium, calcium, vitamin A, vitamin E and dietary fibre) and food groups (vegetables and meat) than those without impaired dentition, after adjusting for potential confounding factors (Iwasaki et al. 2016).

These research findings indicate a likely bidirectional relationship between poor oral function and low number of teeth, on the one hand, and inadequate and poor-quality diet and malnutrition, on the other. Older adults with poor oral function are likely to have a less nutritious diet and poor nutritional status, and the reverse is also true: malnourished older adults are likely to have poor oral function.

Maintaining good oral function is therefore an essential key to longevity. However, there is currently insufficient evidence from longitudinal studies, and in most studies oral function has not been assessed comprehensively enough, so there is a need for additional high-quality studies to further our understanding of this connection.

Recently, the concept of 'oral frailty' has been introduced by Tanaka et al. (2017). According to the Japan Dental Association (JDA), oral frailty presents as a series of phenomena and processes characterized by vulnerable oral health status due to age-related changes in oral health indicators (number of teeth, oral hygiene, oral functions). It is accompanied by a decreased interest in oral health and decreased physical and mental reserve capacity, which can lead to deterioration in eating function, potentially resulting in physical and mental disorders (JDA 2019).

2.6   Assessment of oral health of older adults

2.6.1   Nutrition and diet

Nutrition assessment of older people can be implemented in dental settings by measuring body weight and body mass index (BMI) in order to monitor weight loss rate. Weight loss of 5% in a month or 10% in 6 months is considered to be a sign of possible undernutrition. Calf circumference is another useful measure (Kubo et al. 2009). Dental professionals can also monitor the nutrient (particularly energy and protein) and water consumption of patients. They can also ask about patients' appetite and the reasons for loss of appetite. Protein intake usually decreases in the later stages of life, and protein deficiency is a primary cause of frailty and sarcopenia. Therefore, it is important to maintain and restore appetite and food diversity by maintaining and restoring oral function. Assessment of food diversity is usually performed via the dietary variety score (DVS). The DVS assesses the daily intake of 10 different foods, and a higher score is thought to indicate a higher intake of protein and other nutrients. Nutrition screening of hospital inpatients can be performed using the subject global assessment (SGA) as a subjective evaluation method. The SGA consists of simple interview questions and physical assessments, making it practical to implement with a wide range of age groups and on an ongoing basis. In addition, the Mini Nutritional Assessment® (MNA®) is a subjective evaluation tool for use with older people aged 65 and over, and there is also a short form (MNA®-SF) that is commonly used (Rubenstein et al. 2001).

2.6.2   Assessment of residential environment, family, exercise, health literacy, social activity and economic situation

Older people are more likely to be affected by psychological problems and their social environment, so they need to be evaluated from the perspective of psychological and social frailty. Therefore, in addition to the physical functions of daily living, it is important for oral health professionals to be aware of patients' living environment. Specifically, living environment information that is relevant to oral function management includes: the residential environment, the presence or absence of family members, daily exercise habits, health literacy (access to and ability to make use of health-related information), social connectedness and participation, economic status, and geographical distance and accessibility of oral health services. For older people requiring long-term care, oral health professionals need to coordinate and cooperate with care managers, counsellors, and family caregivers to ensure that sufficient daily oral care can be continuously provided.

2.6.3   Assessment of oral function

When evaluating oral function, it is important to consider the purpose of the evaluation based on the general health condition and daily activities of the subject, to select the appropriate evaluation methods and to conduct the evaluation using standardized, evidence-based techniques. In addition, it is important not to rely on the results of a single evaluation, but to obtain a comprehensive picture of the overall decline of oral function by considering multiple test results in the aggregate.

The oral function of older people is closely related to general health condition and lifestyle (Fukai et al. 2022). Therefore, when evaluating oral function, it is important to take these factors into consideration. This section will provide an outline of oral function evaluation methods that can be used either during dental checkups or in other settings such as outpatient care, elderly care homes or home dental care. From the viewpoint of oral function management, all of these settings are part of an integrated and ongoing process, so a variety of evaluation methods must be integrated into a comprehensive assessment that is tailored to each patient (JDA 2019).

2.6.4   General health and lifestyle factors

In order to develop and select appropriate evaluation methods and interpret the results, it is important to understand the general health and lifestyle factors that are relevant to oral functions. For example, as the elderly often have multiple morbidities, it is important to review the case history and be aware of which diseases the patient has and which medications they are on. Some diseases (e.g. cerebrovascular disease and dementia) and drugs (e.g. for hypertension and depression) may affect oral functions in specific ways. It is also important to be aware of the patient's consciousness level and cognitive function, as patients with cognitive decline often experience a reduction in masticatory function as well as difficulty eating and communicating their thoughts and feelings. Vital signs must be assessed before oral function evaluations begin, and in some cases during the evaluation. For example, if blood oxygen levels are low, there may be a risk of aspiration during the swallowing function test. A patient's posture and physical mobility may also have a limiting effect on some oral functions, so these factors should be observed and noted before beginning the evaluation. Muscle strength (as measured by grip strength) is another factor that is closely related to oral functions, particularly swallowing. Respiratory disease is common among the elderly, and those with declining respiratory function and weakened cough reflex are likely also to experience oral function symptoms such as dysphagia. It is especially important to be aware of the patient's diet and nutrition, which have a strong bidirectional relationship with oral function. Declining oral function is one of the causes of low nutrition, which in turn causes reduced body weight, sarcopenia and frailty. These in turn cause declining oral function, completing the vicious cycle. Finally, the living environment of the patient should also be noted, as family members, daily routines and location of residence can all have an effect on oral function and care. Of particular importance is whether the person lives alone and whether sufficient care can be provided by family members or other professional or non-professional caregivers.

2.6.5 Diseases and medications

As older people often have multiple diseases, dental professionals should check patients' general medical history, including the current status of any ongoing conditions or diseases. When treating patients with cardiovascular or respiratory diseases, care must be taken when extracting teeth and/or performing other procedures involving bleeding. Diseases such as cerebrovascular disease and dementia are known to cause loss of oral function, so it is useful for dentists to be aware of these conditions. Furthermore, when dental care is performed on such patients, it is necessary to communicate and cooperate with the patient's physician. Dentists must also be aware of their patients' medications, as older people are likely to be taking multiple medications. If it is difficult elicit accurate medical information directly from the patient, reviewing the patients' medications usually provides a good indication of the diseases for which they are being treated. Additionally, some drugs affect oral function by causing dry mouth or involuntary movements. In particular, antipsychotic medications may contribute to dysphagia by weakening the swallowing and cough reflexes. The method and frequency of medication administration should also be noted.

2.6.6 Level of consciousness and cognitive function

Consciousness refers to alertness and cognition, with the brain stem controlling the former and the cerebral cortex controlling the latter. If either one or both of them declines, there will be a loss of consciousness. The Glasgow Coma Scale (GCS) is the most commonly used assessment of consciousness level. In dental settings, however, professionals are more likely to use the Mini Mental State Examination (MMSE), which assesses cognitive function when dementia is suspected. In general, dementia is suspected if the MMSE score is 23 points or lower. If the MMSE score is between 24 and 27, mild cognitive impairment (MCI) is suspected. However, the MMSE score alone is not a sufficient basis for a diagnosis. Diagnosis of dementia and MCI requires a comprehensive judgment by a physician based on interviews, physical examination and imaging, along with a number of cognitive function tests. Another assessment tool used to determine the severity of dementia is the Clinical Dementia Rating (CDR). The CDR provides a multi-faceted assessment of cognitive function based on behavioural observations and information from caregivers. Alzheimer's disease is progressive, so the functional assessment staging (FAST) method, a classification system used to assess the stage of cognitive decline, is also useful. It is important for dental professionals to notice the connection between oral function decline and cognitive decline (Naito 2015; Motokawa et al. 2021).

2.6.7 Vital signs

Vital signs are indicators of the body's most important life-sustaining functions that can be measured and monitored. They include blood pressure, heart rate, respiratory rate, body temperature and consciousness. In particular, breathing and circulation, which are the essential requirements of life, are often monitored by blood oxygen saturation (SpO2), blood pressure, heart rate and electrocardiogram. Older people generally have low reserve capacity, so monitoring vital signs is one way for oral health professionals to be aware of how the treatment can inflict stress on these patients. In this sense, monitoring vital signs can be seen as a type of risk management activity to prevent the onset of systemic side-effects that can occur during dental examinations.

2.6.8 Activities of daily living and posture

Activities of daily living (ADLs) and posture retention, such as head position and trunk posture, also affect diet and quality of life (QOL), which are related to oral function evaluation. ADLs are largely separated into basic activities and instrumental activities. The Barthel Index and the Functional Independence Measure (FIM) are used to evaluate basic activities of daily living. The former evaluates whether a person *can do* certain activities, and the latter evaluates whether a person *actually does* certain activities. These measures can be used to determine the level of care needed. The Instrumental Activities of Daily Living (IADL) scale measures more complex and labour-requiring activities, such as using the telephone, shopping and doing housework. On all of these scales, a higher score indicates greater independence. These measures can be important in oral function evaluation because they are related to walking, movement, posture, oral health behaviour and diet.

2.6.9 Muscle strength and paralysis

Knowing the muscle strength of older patients, as well as whether or not they have paralysis, is very important because this aspect of the patient's physical condition are related not only to the prevention of frailty and sarcopenia, but also to oral function. For example, in order to assess swallowing function, it is important to be aware of differences between the left and right sides of the body, particularly in terms of trunk muscle strength, neck muscle strength, and facial and tongue muscle movement, which are important for spitting and swallowing. The simplest and most practical strength assessment is grip strength. In general, a grip strength assessment is conducted twice with each hand, and the better result is recorded. In Japan, low muscle strength is suspected when the grip strength is lower than 26 kg in men or 18 kg in women (Chen et al. 2014). If grip strength measuring equipment is not available, a rough assessment can be obtained by shaking the patient's hand.

2.6.10 Breathing and vocal capacity

Respiratory function and cough reflexes generally decline with age, often in conjunction with respiratory diseases such as chronic obstructive pulmonary disease. Therefore, from the viewpoint of preventing aspiration pneumonia, oral health professionals should assess the breathing of older patients. Particular attention is warranted with patients who have previously developed aspiration pneumonia. In addition, pneumonia is often asymptomatic in older people, so dental professionals should pay attention even to less obvious symptoms such as slight fever, increased sputum production, anorexia and a decrease in ADLs.

Respiratory function can be evaluated by assessing maximum phonation time (MPT) of vowel sounds. There is a gender difference, but in healthy elderly people, normal MPT is considered to be in the range of 10–15 seconds (Hagio 2004). Another sign of respiratory function decline is chronic hoarseness, which may take a variety of forms and be caused by glottal or nasal closure, so dental professionals should take notice if patients present with abnormal vocal characteristics.

2.6.11 Assessment of the oral environment

Assessment of the oral environment involves assessing the state of a patient's oral hygiene, saliva, teeth, gums, mucous membrane, etc. These aspects of the oral environment influence and are influenced by the various movements and forces of the oral components (jaws, tongue, etc.) The vital oral functions of chewing and swallowing are the result of the integration of these components, movements and forces.

Assessing the oral environment requires two different types of assessment: one for oral hygiene and saliva, and another for teeth, gums and the oral mucous membrane. An oral assessment tool that can be used to comprehensively assess the oral environment is also useful.

2.6.11.1 Dental plaque and tongue coating

Poor oral hygiene in older patients can cause aspiration pneumonia and oral infections due to an abnormal increase in microorganisms in the oral cavity, which can also cause bad breath. Oral hygiene is assessed by measuring the degree of plaque adhesion and tongue coating.

There are three measurements commonly used to assess the degree of plaque adhesion, all of which rely on dyeing: Plaque Control Record (PCR), Debris Index, and Plaque Index. However, there is a greater degree of tooth loss in older people, and plaque may accumulate on the mucous membrane as well as dentures, so it is difficult to obtain an accurate measurement via dyeing procedures alone, especially in long-term care recipients.

Tongue coating is also a useful indicator because it can be assessed even in toothless jaws, and it is, like plaque, a measure of oral hygiene. The Tongue Coating Index (TCI) is used for this purpose. The TCI involves dividing the dorsal surface of the tongue into several small areas and evaluating the degree of coating on each area with a three-step scale (0, no coating; 1, thin coating; 2, thick coating). The scores can then be added together to arrive at a total TCI score. Another method is Shimizu's method (Shimizu et al. 2007), which involves dividing the dorsum of the tongue into nine parts and then assessing the degree of coating in a more fine-grained manner. When assessing tongue coating, the clinician must also pay attention to the colour of the coating. It is usually white, so care should be taken to distinguish it from pseudomembranous candidiasis (thrush). The coating may also appear yellow depending on the thickness of the coating or the patient's diet. If the colour is black, it is often due to black hairy tongue, a condition caused by microbial substitution due to the long-term administration of antibacterial drugs and adrenocortical hormones.

2.6.11.2 Dry mouth and saliva flow

Saliva is normally secreted at a rate of 1–1.5 L/day, and it plays an important role in the preservation of the oral environment. For this, reason, it is important to assess the amount and quality of elderly patients' saliva, as well as the degree of dryness and flow.

Oral dryness is diagnosed on the basis of subjective symptoms such as abnormal dryness in the oral cavity, declining fit and stability of dentures, discomfort when using dentures, and weakening of the mucous membrane. Due to a decrease in the amount of saliva, the movement of the tongue, lips and cheeks becomes restricted; chewing, swallowing and conversation become difficult; and the sense of taste becomes dull. As a result, the enjoyment of eating decreases. Causes of dry mouth include systemic diseases, medication side-effects, ageing and decreased oral motor function.

2.6.11.3 Halitosis

Halitosis (bad breath) can be caused by plaque in the oral cavity, coated tongue, or decreased saliva flow. When the patient's mouth cannot be opened due to clenching or resistance to care, bad breath can be a useful sign of poor oral conditions such as plaque and coated tongue.

2.6.11.4 Level of independence in performance of daily oral cleaning

When evaluating oral hygiene behaviour, caregivers should assess the extent to which patients can independently perform daily oral cleaning (oral care-related ADLs). In other words, there is a need to assess whether patients are self-supporting or require partial or full assistance with regard to oral hygiene, gargling, dentures, and so on.

2.6.11.5 Assessment of teeth, dentures, gums, mucous membranes, jawbones and jaw joints

Dentists should conduct regular assessment of dental caries, periodontal disease and oral mucosal diseases, and they should also record the number of remaining functional teeth and the presence and type of dentures.

Dentists should also examine patients for dental diseases that are prevalent among the elderly, such as tooth fractures, cracked or chipped teeth, root caries, dental implants, oral candidiasis, stomatitis, bisphosphonate-related osteonecrosis of the jaw (BRONJ) and need of urgent dental treatment.

2.6.11.6 Comprehensive assessment of the oral environment

The two most commonly used comprehensive oral assessments tools are the Revised Oral Assessment Guide (ROAG) (Andersson et al. 2002) and the Oral Health Assessment Tool (OHAT) (Chalmers et al. 2005). ROAG is used to assess oral hygiene status in order to prevent stomatitis in cancer patients. OHAT is used evaluate the oral environment, including denture fit, of older patients. These assessment tools are useful for sharing information about patients' oral condition among multiple professionals who are responsible for day-to-day oral care, such as nurses and speech therapists.

2.6.11.7 Assessment of integrated oral function

Integrated oral function refers not to the function of individual oral organs, but to the integrated set of functions that occur in the oral cavity, such as chewing, swallowing, conversation and non-verbal communication (facial expression). Healthy oral function depends not only on a healthy oral environment and individual oral functions, but also on integrated oral function. The following sections outline methods for evaluating integrated oral function, with a particular focus on chewing and swallowing functions, because these two functions are most closely related to dental care. Chewing function and swallowing function are explained separately in the following sections, but it is important to be aware that they are actually integrated as a single process: eating. However, it is possible to have normal chewing function while also having difficulty swallowing.

2.6.11.8 Assessment of mastication

Older people often experience a decline in chewing and swallowing function due to senescence and/or various diseases. Declining chewing and swallowing function can, in turn, lead to aspiration pneumonia. Therefore, healthy eating habits and the maintenance of chewing function are essential elements of elderly health and well-being. To that end, oral health professionals need to be proficient in using a variety of assessment methods to assess and monitor patients' masticatory and swallowing function.

2.6.11.9 Observation of the act of eating

The chewing process begins when food is brought into the oral cavity and ends with the act of swallowing. The act of chewing itself involves formation and transport of a mass of food material suitable for swallowing by repeatedly biting and grinding the food while mixing it with saliva. Chewing function can be assessed by observing people in the act of eating. Once normal chewing has been observed, chewing function problems can be identified by visual comparison.

The eating process can be divided into five stages. The first three stages are the cognitive, pre-paratory and oral cavity (chewing) stages. The last two stages are the pharyngeal and oesophageal stages of swallowing.

2.6.11.10 Assessment of consumable foods

The simplest way to assess chewing function is to ask a patient which foods he or she is able to eat. With older patients, in particular, it is important to ask them on a daily basis which foods and food states (whole, cut, mashed, etc.) they are able to eat, and to record and notice how their responses change over time. Another method is to ask patients to fill out a daily questionnaire in which they identify the types of food they are able to ingest. Several such ingestible food questionnaires have been developed (Sato et al. 1988).

2.6.11.11 Chewing and grinding ability

A quantitative method of chewing function assessment is to measure the concentration of glucose extracted from chewing gummy candies.

2.6.11.12 Food mixing ability

Another assessment of chewing ability focuses on the ability to mix bits of food with saliva in the mouth. In this assessment, the patient chews a piece of gum 60 times (one bite per second) and then discharges it from the oral cavity. The colour of the gum is then observed and recorded visually (using a colour scale), or it can be assessed with a spectrophotometer.

2.6.11.13 Ability to form boluses (salivary masses)

Recent studies have shown that the ability to form boluses can be assessed by using a video endo-scope to directly observe the state of the bolus in the pharynx during swallowing (Abe et al. 2011; Fukatsu et al. 2015).

2.6.11.14 Assessment of swallowing function

2.6.11.14.1 Observe the act of eating   Like chewing, the most basic form of swallowing assessment is observing a person while they are eating. Once an expert knows what the normal mechanism of swallowing looks like, they can then look for abnormalities in the swallowing function of a patient. Of the five stages of eating mentioned earlier, the practitioner will focus primarily on visual assessment of the oral (chewing) and pharyngeal (swallowing) stages. They will check not only the swallowing function, but also the breathing function.

2.6.11.14.2 Subjective assessment   Decreased swallowing function refers to the pre-dysphagia stage, where swallowing function has begun to decrease with age. EAT-10 (the 10-item Eating Assessment Tool) (Belafsky et al. 2008) is a screening tool used to subjectively evaluate swallowing function. EAT-10 consists of 10 questions and a score of 3 or more signifies that swallowing function is impaired.

2.6.11.14.3 Screening tests   Screening tests are often performed for the purpose of obtaining information before a more thorough examination such as an endoscopy, or for the purpose of establishing standards of normal function. Note that in patients who are currently able to eat, the information obtained from observation of eating is often more useful than screening tests. However, in patients who are unable to eat, screening tests can be invaluable in order to determine the necessity of a thorough examination or whether oral intake can be resumed. Simple screening tests for swallowing function include the Repetitive Saliva Swallowing Test (RSST), the Modified Water Swallowing Test (MWST), the Food Test (FT) and cervical auscultation.

The RSST is a test in which the patient is asked to swallow as many times as possible in 30 seconds, and the result is recorded. If the patient is able to swallow fewer than three times, dysphagia (aspiration) is suspected. It is easier and safer than other tests because the patient is just swallowing their own saliva. However, it may be difficult to conduct this test if the patient is unable to follow instructions or if the patient has a dry mouth.

The MWST is a test in which 3 ml of cold water is placed in the oral cavity and swallowed, and the swallowing function of the pharynx is assessed by noting the presence or absence of the swallowing reflex, the presence or absence of a coughing response, the respiratory condition, and presence or absence of a wet-hoarse voice. These criteria are used to record the result, which is on a five-point scale. This test is easy to conduct even if the patient cannot understand the dentist's instructions well.

The FT involves having the patient swallow 3–4 g of pudding and then assessing the swallowing function in the same way as the MWST and also noting any pudding remaining in the oral cavity. It is easier to detect oral disorders with this test than with the MWST. A disadvantage of using the MWST and FT to detect swallowing function disorders is that they rely heavily on the presence or absence of coughing, but it is possible to have swallowing problems that are not accompanied by coughing.

Cervical auscultation assesses the swallowing function in the pharynx by using a stethoscope to listen to the patient's breathing and swallowing sounds before and after swallowing. This is an easy and non-invasive auxiliary method that is often used in conjunction with other tests. Multiple screening tests should be used in order to improve the accuracy of the assessment.

2.6.11.14.4 *Detailed examination*

Swallowing is a function that occurs inside the oral cavity and the pharynx, so it is difficult to observe from the outside. Therefore, in cases where a more precise assessment is required for final diagnosis, it is necessary to perform an image inspection using videofluoroscopy (VF) or videoendoscopy (VE). In VF, a series of swallows are indirectly observed by X-ray. The first stages of the swallowing process, from introduction of food into the oral cavity to transportation of food material to the stomach, can be observed by lateral and frontal X-ray images, and aspiration and gastro-oesophageal reflux during swallowing can also be observed. However, VF requires the use of simulated food containing barium, which may not necessarily reflect daily eating function. VE, on the other hand, involves direct observation of the pharynx using a nasopharyngeal endoscope. This device is highly portable and can therefore be carried out by the bedside or even at the patient's home or a nursing care facility, so the advantage of using this method is that the patient's normal daily eating and swallowing habits can be accurately observed. VF and VE are mutually complementary imaging methods that must be used with a full understanding of their respective characteristics.

2.6.11.14.5 *Comprehensive evaluation*

When considering how to proceed with treatment of dysphagia in older patients, it is useful to make a comprehensive determination of the level of clinical severity based on the results of the various observations, screening tests and detailed examinations of swallowing function described earlier. Determining the overall level of swallowing function disorder in this way would allow for easy dissemination to and understanding by all healthcare professionals involved in caring for a given patient. It would also make it easy for all involved to see whether the patient's condition is stable or changing. For example, Saito's dysphagia clinical severity scale (Dysphagia Severity Scale, DSS) (Nishimura et al. 2015) allows for comprehensive evaluation of a patient's ability to swallow based on a seven-level system.

2.7   Dementia and oral healthcare in dental clinics

Dementia is the leading cause of dependency and it is inevitable that the burden of dementia will increase in an ageing society. Dental patients often visit their dentist for a long period of time. It is therefore important that dentists and dental team are concerned with the prevention of cognitive decline. This section describes some evidence for the prevention of cognitive decline, based on Japanese guidelines for the dental treatment of people with dementia (Fukai et al. 2019).

2.7.1   The effect of dental maintenance on the delay and prevention of dementia onset

It is likely that regular dental maintenance has an indirect effect on the delay and prevention of the onset of dementia. Regular and continuous dental maintenance is effective in preventing oral diseases and maintaining oral function. This, in turn, supports healthy social functioning, which likely contributes to delaying the onset of dementia. However, few studies have investigated this relationship over the long term, so there is currently insufficient evidence to make a strong claim of effectiveness.

Dental visitation gives people living with dementia a reason and opportunity to leave home and interact with others. In addition, maintaining good oral health through regular dental intervention supports nutrition intake, which itself contributes to prevention of cognitive decline.

A great deal of research has been conducted on the relationship between diet and dementia, revealing that regular dietary guidance is probably effective in delaying or preventing the onset of dementia. A large portion of the population receives regular and continuing dietary guidance at their local dental clinic, so this represents a significant and effective public health approach to dementia prevention.

Older people often experience a decline in chewing and swallowing function, but for people living with dementia, there are many additional factors that negatively affect food intake and nutrition. Factors include the type and stage of dementia, the specific behavioural and psychological symptoms being experienced, the severity of interruption of ADLs, the side-effects of medication, and other environmental factors. Moreover, the diversity of food consumed by older people tends to be limited, and this phenomenon is particularly pronounced among those living alone.

Recent studies have reported that diet and nutrition are highly associated with cognitive decline and dementia. Therefore, dental professionals who have been well trained in dental clinics have great potential to contribute to the maintenance of cognitive function of older patients by providing regular and high-quality dietary instruction.

In developed countries, the rate and frequency of dental visitation are higher than those of medical check-ups and treatment. In Japan, for example, half of the population reports having visited a dentist in the past year (Fukai 2019) and most people have easy access to dental care. Therefore, providing dietary guidance in dental clinics has the potential to be a powerful public health approach to reducing cognitive decline among the population at large. For this reason, dental clinics should make greater effort to develop and enhance their dietary instruction content and procedures.

2.7.2   Does tooth loss prevention and prevention of oral function decline at dental clinics help delay or prevent the onset of dementia?

There is evidence that tooth loss prevention and prevention of oral function decline are highly likely to delay or prevent dementia.

Preventing tooth loss prevents cognitive decline and the onset of dementia, and the reverse is also likely true. The evidence reviewed in this chapter consists only of observational research, which is considered weaker than interventional research. However, there are serious ethical limitations on conducting interventional research on tooth loss (it would involve extracting teeth), so the best way to strengthen the evidence of this relationship is to accumulate and analyse evidence from a wide variety of countries and regions with differing socioeconomic status, healthcare systems, and so on.

Severe periodontal disease leads to loss of teeth, resulting in a decrease in oral function, including chewing function. The reviews described in this chapter have investigated the relationship between oral health and dementia. In particular, in recent years, many reports have revealed a link between periodontal disease and tooth loss, on the one hand, and the onset of cognitive decline and dementia on the other. Therefore, oral hygiene care and treatment for the prevention of tooth loss and periodontal disease is likely to contribute to preventing and delaying the onset of dementia and reducing its severity.

In addition, given that periodontal disease is also a major cause of tooth loss, there are likely two pathways by which oral health prevention contributes to the prevention and delay of cognitive decline. The first is a direct path, whereby periodontal disease prevention itself delays/prevents the onset of cognitive decline and dementia, and the second is an indirect path, whereby periodontal disease prevention activities prevent tooth loss, which in turn delays or prevents cognitive decline.

2.7.3   What barriers must be overcome in order to prevent dental disease and decline of oral health function in people with cognitive decline?

A limited amount of research shows that the effectiveness of dental disease prevention in people with dementia depends on the continuing and dedicated support of the person's family or other caregivers, but further research in this area is needed.

When cognitive function decreases, it becomes difficult to learn new things, but it is possible to continue performing the oral cleaning habits that have been previously acquired and practised throughout the person's life. However, sufficient dental plaque removal becomes gradually more difficult, which leads to worsening oral hygiene status. The onset and progression of cognitive decline often require the daily support of family members and/or caregivers in order to maintain oral health behaviours.

It has been suggested that the implementation of long-term oral care interventions can help to prevent the need for long-term nursing care among elderly people, and that it is also effective in improving their enthusiasm for life while maintaining and improving oral functions.

In addition to establishing good oral health behaviours while still healthy (before the onset of dementia), it is also necessary to involve family members and/or professional caregivers (ideally dental health professionals) in the maintenance of oral health during the early stages of dementia (Sumi et al. 2012). This means that screening and early detection can have a great effect on maintenance of oral health.

There is still a relative scarcity of research in this area, so much more research is needed before consensus can be reached on the importance of dental health support for those living with dementia.

2.7.4   How should dental treatment and maintenance plans be adjusted for people with different levels of cognitive decline?

As dementia progresses, it becomes more and more difficult to adapt to changes in the surrounding environment. Because the oral cavity is a sensitive part of the body, dental patients with dementia often show strong resistance to dental care or oral care. In order to create an environment in which dental care is easier to accept, it is useful to begin by providing opportunities for the patient to experience short, low-pressure, low-pain experiences with dental professionals and dental intervention (Fiske et al. 2006).

As cognitive decline progresses, it becomes more and more difficult for people with dementia to manage their own complex oral healthcare routines. It is important for dentists to understand this and explain to the family or caregivers that dental treatment plans may have to be adjusted in consideration of the patient's ability to maintain the necessary daily care routine.

Dental professionals must consider how to effectively and safely administer dental care to patients with cognitive impairment, and they must also be aware of the progressive nature of this condition (Gordon 1988). They must collect and assimilate information from medical personnel, nursing care workers and family members in order to determine whether cognitive decline is present or not (Gordon 1988). Dentists also can and should contribute to the prevention and control of dementia and cognitive decline as part of a cooperative, multi-professional team.

Comprehensive reviews and government guidelines in both Japan (Fukai et al. 2019) and the UK (National Health Service England 2016; Batchelor 2017) have recommended that dental care should be tailored to each patient's cognitive function level. In order to do this, dental professionals must first identify the patient's current stage of cognitive decline (mild, moderate or severe) and then adjust their dental treatment plan accordingly. This is extremely important, as the dental care provided at the earlier stages can slow the progression of cognitive decline itself (due to influencing the patient's eating function and behaviour).

2.7.4.1 Mild

At this stage there are few obstacles to regular dental care and treatment, as patients are still relatively aware of their own oral status and can voice their complaints (Gordon 1988). However, dental professionals must recognize that treatment will become progressively more difficult in the future. Complex prosthetic procedures can also be conducted, assuming the patient's family and/or caregivers can assist with the patient's daily oral hygiene. Considering the progressive nature of dementia, prevention of subsequent periodontal disease becomes particularly important at this stage, so dental professionals need to move beyond the treatment-only paradigm and provide advice and information on the prevention of oral disease to these patients, their families and their caregivers.

2.7.4.2 Moderate

At this stage, patients are more likely to reject dental treatment due to difficulty understanding the explanation provided by the dental professional. Special consideration and/or arrangements may be needed, particularly for treatments that inflict a psychological burden, such as procedures that are extremely painful or take a long time to complete. For example, the patient may need to be given more breaks than usual, or more anaesthesia. When deciding on a treatment plan, the patient often has trouble making decisions independently, so the course of treatment may be determined by considering how cooperative the patient is, the dental care needs of the patient, other existing health conditions, and the social support system available to the patient (Batchelor 2017). If possible, the treatment plan should be carefully explained to the patient's family and informed consent obtained.

2.7.4.3 Severe

At the stage of severe cognitive decline, communication between patient and dental professional becomes very difficult or impossible, and the cognitive decline is very often accompanied by a decline in physical function. When deciding on a dental treatment plan for these individuals, the dentist must obtain information about their daily life from their family or other caregivers and also listen to the family's preferences and consider their living arrangements and caregiving plans. In cases where complete and/or ideal treatment is deemed difficult, the dentist should implement a course of treatment that helps the patient maintain basic oral function but requires minimal intervention while prioritizing the patient's comfort and QOL (Batchelor 2017).

2.8   Oral healthcare systems: community-based and clinical-based approach

Central to confronting the challenges of healthy ageing is prevention of ageing-related functional decline. This means that the goal for healthy ageing is to maintain functional ability and prevent its decline as much as possible. In both community settings and individual contexts, it is necessary to take a person-centred approach, which involves a new emphasis on assessing and screening older people for decline in functional ability (motor ability, eating ability, cognitive ability, etc.) in addition to the current focus on disease detection.

In order to achieve a healthy ageing society, policies focusing on the assessment and maintenance of oral functions are needed. An approach centred on the assessment and screening of the oral function of older individuals and the subsequent multi-sectoral response would mark a shift towards a person-centred approach that is based on interprofessional cooperation (Fukai et al. 2022).

What challenges must be overcome to support the oral health needs of an ageing society? Oral healthcare systems (OHCSs) seek to maintain the oral health and oral function of a population via three methods: oral health promotion, prevention, and disease control and management. A country's national health agenda affects the degree of priority given to each of these three methods, and that distribution of priority in turn determines what services are provided, which population groups are served, funding and research priorities and data acquisition. OHCSs must adapt when confronted with demographic changes such as the increasingly ageing population, although they have traditionally been slow to adapt. Figure 2.7 identifies some of the challenges facing OHCSs around the world as they seek to adapt to demographic changes [World Dental Federation (FDI) OHAP Task Team 2018]. Some countries have already overcome some of the challenges, and the experiences of such countries show that effective solutions can be found and implemented if priorities are clarified and supported.

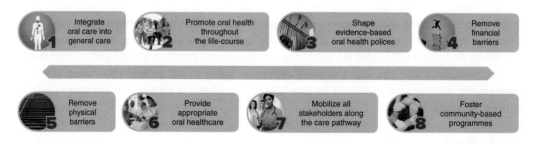

Figure 2.7   Eight different fields of action for stakeholders. *Source:* © FDI World Dental Federation / https://www.fdiworlddental.org/roadmap-healthy-ageing/ accessed 5 September 2023.

Table 2.2 Stakeholders for establishment of an oral healthcare system.

- Policymakers and governments
- FDI World Dental Federation
- National dental associations
- Dentists and dental teams
- Health professionals (e.g. physicians, nurses, nurse assistants)
- Public health professionals
- Research and academia
- Media (press, television, social media)
- Patients and their families

In order for countries to adapt their OHCSs to address the needs of ageing populations, a coalition of stakeholders is required. The roadmap in Table 2.2 lists the stakeholders who can be called upon to contribute to improving the OHCS, each based on their own area of expertise. The roadmap itself can be viewed on the OHAP Task Team project on the FDI website (https://www.fdiworlddental.org/roadmap-healthy-ageing). The challenges are policy and advocacy, provision of care, education and training, monitoring and surveillance, evidence and research, and communication and information.

According to FDI OHAP, these stakeholders can act via eight different fields of action (FDI OHAP Task Team 2018) in order to achieve the implementation of an OHCS that meets the needs of older adults. In Figure 2.7, the actions and roles of each stakeholder are presented. With this resource in hand, therefore, each stakeholder group can easily identify, in a concrete manner, how they can contribute to the maintenance and improvement of oral health in older adults. It also positions each stakeholder's role within the context of the contributions of other stakeholders, showing how each stakeholder group complements the contributions of others.

Oral healthcare systems need to be reformed to allow older people to lead lives of purpose and dignity. The most needed reforms are as follows: integrating oral health into overall health; employing a life-course approach that accounts for common risk factors; implementing a community-based approach; integrating and drawing on the strengths of all stakeholders; sharing of tasks and responsibilities among stakeholders; ensuring accessibility to care (both financial and physical); and establishing an enabling environment. To achieve this, the four-step approach recommended by Fukai et al. (2018) can be employed. This approach integrates and builds on the contributions of each stakeholder group to achieve the gradual adoption of oral healthcare systems that meet the needs of elderly populations and promote improvement in their oral health and oral health-related quality of life.

2.9 Conclusion

Restoring oral function in older people is important for the prevention of frailty and for preventing and reducing dependence on long-term care. In addition, the risk of oral diseases continues throughout all life stages, so dental professionals are likely to care for patients frequently, regularly and over a long period of time. This means that dental professionals are uniquely positioned to notice small, gradual changes in the physical and mental condition, including the oral function, of older patients.

In order to prevent non-communicable diseases and frailty, which are highly associated with oral health, there is a need for communities and dental institutions to collaborate to implement public health programmes which include assessment and screening and are based on the principle of inter-professional cooperation and driven by national policy.

References

Abe, R., Furuya, J., & Suzuki, T. (2011). Videoendoscopic measurement of food bolus formation for quantitative evaluation of masticatory function. *J Prosthodont Res*, 55(3), 171–178.

Andersson, P., Hallberg, I. R., & Renvert, S. (2002). Inter-rater reliability of an oral assessment guide for elderly patients residing in a rehabilitation ward. *Spec Care Dentist*, 22(5), 181–6.

Batchelor, P. (2017). *Dementia-Friendly Dentistry –Good Practice Guidelines*. London, UK: Faculty of General Dental Practice.

Belafsky, P. C., Mouadeb, D. A., Rees, C. J. et al. (2008). Validity and reliability of the Eating Assessment Tool EAT-1. *Ann Otol Rhinol Laryngol*, 117, 919–924.

Chalmers, J. M., King, P. L., Spencer, A. J., Wright, F. A., & Carter, K. D. (2005). The oral health assessment tool – Validity and reliability. *Aust Dent J*, 50, 191–199.

Chen, L. K., Liu, L. K., Woo, J. et al. (2014Feb). Sarcopenia in Asia: consensus report of the Asian Working Group for Sarcopenia. *J Am Med Dir Assoc*, 15(2), 95–101.

Chen, L. K., Woo, J., Assantachai, P. et al. (2020). 2019 Consensus update on sarcopenia diagnosis and treatment. *J Am Med Dir Assoc*, 21(3), 300–307.e2.

Cruz-Jentoft, A. J., Baeyens, J. P., Bauer, J. M. et al., European Working Group on Sarcopenia in Older People. (2010 July). Sarcopenia: European consensus on definition and diagnosis: Report of the European working group on sarcopenia in older people. *Age Ageing*, 39(4), 412–423.

Dent, E., Morley, J. E., Cruz-Jentoft, A. J. et al. (2019). Physical frailty: ICFSR International clinical practice guidelines for identification and management. *J Nutr Health Aging*, 23(9), 771–787.

FDI Oral Health for an Ageing Population Task Team. (2018). *Roadmap for Healthy Ageing*. Geneva: FDI. https://www.fdiworlddental.org/roadmap-healthy-ageing (accessed 13 May 2024).

Fiske, J., Frenkel, H., Griffiths, J., & Jones, V. (2006). Guidelines for the development of local standards of oral health care for people with dementia. *Gerodontology*, 23 Suppl 1, 5–32.

Fried, L.P., Tangen, C.M., Walston, J. et al. & Cardiovascular Health Study Collaborative Research Group. (2001). Frailty in older adults: evidence for a phenotype. *J Gerontol A Biol Sci Med Sci*, 56(3), M146–156.

Fukai, K., Dartevelle, S., Jones, J. (2022). Oral health for healthy ageing: a people-centred and function-focused approach. *Int Dent*, 72(4S), S2–S4.

Fukai, K., Yoshihara, A., Ogawa, H. et al.(2019). *Ninchisho No Hitono Shikachiryo Guideline [The Dental-care Guideline for the Older People with Dementia]*. Tokyo: Ishiyaku Publishers Inc, 52–79 (in Japanese).

Fukai, K. (2019). Oral health for healthy aging society-evidence and health policy. *JJHEP*, 27(4), 360–368.

Fukai, K., Hori, K., Benz, C. et al. & FDI OHAP Task Team. (2018). Oral Health for Ageing Populations Roadmap For Healthy Ageing. Geneva: FDI. https://www.fdiworlddental.org/sites/default/files/2020–11/ohap-2018-roadmap_ageing.pdf (accessed 13 May 2024).

Fukatsu, H., Nohara, K., Kotani, Y. et al. (2015). Endoscopic evaluation of food bolus formation and its relationship with the number of chewing cycles. *J Oral Rehab*, 42(8), 580–587.

Gatz, M., Mortimer, J. A., Fratiglioni, L. et al. (2006). Potentially modifiable risk factors for dementia in identical twins. *Alzheimers Dement*, 2(2), 110–117.

Glick, M., Williams, D.M., Kleinman, D.V. et al. (2016). A new definition for oral health developed by the FDI World Dental Federation opens the door to a universal definition of oral health. *Int Dent J*, 66(6), 322–324.

GBD 2017 Oral Disorders Collaborators, Bernabe, E., Marcenes, W., Hernandez, C.R. et al. (2020). Global, regional, and national levels and trends in burden of oral conditions from 1990 to 2017: a systematic analysis for the Global Burden of Disease 2017 study. *J Dent Res*, 99(4), 362–373.

Gordon, S. (1988). Argument in favour of providing dental care for the severely cognitively impaired patient. *Gerodontics*, 4(4), 170–171.

Hagio, Y. (2004). Investigation of the standard voice function value of the elderly. *Koutou*, 16, 111–121.

Igarashi, K., Kikutani, T., & Tamura, F. (2019, Jan 23;). Survey of suspected dysphagia prevalence in home-dwelling older people using the 10-Item Eating Assessment Tool (eAT-10). *PLoS One*, 14(1), e0211040.

Iwao, Y., Shigeishi, H., Takahashi, S. et al. (2019). Improvement of physical and oral function in community-dwelling older people after a 3-month long-term care prevention program including physical exercise, oral health instruction, and nutritional guidance. *Clin Exp Dent Res*, 5(6), 611–619.

Iwasaki, M., Hirano, H., Ohara, Y., & Motokawa, K. (2021Nov). The association of oral function with dietary intake and nutritional status among older adults: latest evidence from epidemiological studies. *Jpn Dent Sci Rev*, 57, 128–137.

Iwasaki, M., Yoshihara, A., Kimura, Y. et al. (2016). Longitudinal relationship of severe periodontitis with cognitive decline in older Japanese. *J Periodontal Res*, 51(5), 681–688.

Japan Dental Association (JDA) (2019). Manual of oral frailty at dental clinics, Tokyo (in Japanese). https://www.jda.or.jp/dentist/oral_frail/pdf/manual_all.pdf (accessed 30 June 2024).

Kassebaum, N.J., Bernabé, E., Dahiya, M. et al. (2014a). Global burden of severe periodontitis in 1990–2010: a systematic review and meta-regression. *J Dent Res*, 93, 1045–1053.

Kassebaum, N.J., Bernabé, E., Dahiya, M. et al. (2014b). Global burden of severe tooth loss: a systematic review and meta-analysis. *J Dent Res*, 93, 20S–28S.

Kassebaum, N.J., Bernabé, E., Dahiya, M. et al. (2015). Global burden of untreated caries: a systematic review and metaregression. *J Dent Res*, 94, 650–658.

Kassebaum, N.J., Smith, A. G. C, Bernabé, E. et al. & GBD 2015 Oral Health Collaborators. (2017). Global, regional, and national prevalence, incidence, and disability-adjusted life years for oral conditions for 195 countries, 1990–2015: a systematic analysis for the global burden of diseases, injuries, and risk factors. *J Dent Res*, 96(4), 380–387.

Kikutani, T., Yoneyama, T., Nishiwaki, K. et al. (2010). Effect of oral care on cognitive function in patients with dementia. *Geriatr Gerontol Int*, 10(4), 327–328.

Kimura, Y., Ogawa, H., Yoshihara, A. et al. (2013). Evaluation of chewing ability and its relationship with activities of daily living, depression, cognitive status and food intake in community-dwelling elderly people. *Geriatr Gerontol Int*, 13, 718–725.

Kubo, A., Yoshimatsu, T., Nishida, Y. (2009). Relation of the maximum calf circumference with albumin and body mass index in elderly cases of chronic hospitalization, *Nippon Ronen Igakkai Zasshi*, 46, 239–243.

Livingston, G., Sommerlad, A., Orgeta, V. et al. (2017). Dementia prevention, intervention, and care. *Lancet*, 390, 2673–2734.

Lourida, I., Soni, M., Thompson-Coon, J. et al. (2013). Mediterranean diet, cognitive function, and dementia: a systematic review. *Epidemiology*, 24(4), 479–489.

Minakuchi, S., Tsuga, K., Ikebe, K et al. (2018). Oral hypofunction in the older population: position paper of the Japanese Society of Gerodontology in 2016. *Gerodontology*, 35(4), 317–324.

Motokawa, K., Mikami, Y., Shirobe, M. et al. (2021). Relationship between chewing ability and nutritional status in Japanese older adults: a cross-sectional study. *Int J Environ Res Public Health*, 18(3), 1216.

MHLW of Japan (2024). Guidelines for health services based on the characteristics of older people (in Japanese). 3rd ed. 2024, Tokyo, MHLW. https://www.mhlw.go.jp/content/001240315.pdf (accessed 8 July 2024).

Naito, M. (2015). Rest/communication and QOL, Japan Dental Association (JDA) (Editor in chief: Fukai K) (2015). The current evidence of dental care and oral health for achieving healthy longevity in an aging society. Tokyo: JDA, pp. 204–213. https://www.jda.or.jp/dentist/program/pdf/world_concgress_2015_evidence_en.pdf (accessed 8 July 2024).

National Health Service England. (2024). *Working Towards Dementia Friendly Dental Practices. Health Education England South East.* https://thamesvalley.hee.nhs.uk/dental-directorate-thames-valley-and-wessex/dementia/ (accessed 8 July 2024).

Nishimura, K., Kagaya, H., Shibata, S. et al. (2015). Accuracy of Dysphagia Severity Scale rating without using videoendoscopic evaluation of swallowing. *Jpn J Compr Rehabil Sci*, 6, 124–128.

Ohara, Y., Yoshida, N., Kono, Y. et al. (2015). Effectiveness of an oral health educational program on community-dwelling older people with xerostomia. *Geriatr Gerontol Int*, l5(4), 48l–489.

Perneczky, R., Wagenpfeil, S., Komossa, K. et al. (2006). Mapping scores onto stages: mini-mental state examination and clinical dementia rating. *Am J Geriatr Psychiatry*,14(2), 139–144.

Pretty, I.A., Ellwood, R.P., Lo, E.C.M. et al. (2014). The Seattle Care Pathway for securing oral health in older patients. *Gerodontology*, 31(1), 77–87.

Rubenstein, L. Z., Harker, J. O, Salvà, A. et al. (2001). Screening for undernutrition in geriatric practice: developing the short-form mini-nutritional assessment (MNA®-SF). *J Gerontol A Biol Sci Med Sci.* 56(6), M366–372.

Sakayori, T., Maki, Y., Hirata, S. et al. (2013). Evaluation of a Japanese "Prevention of Long-term Care" project for the improvement in oral function in the high-risk elderly. *Geriatr Gerontol Int*, 13(2), 451–457.

Sato, Y., Ishida, E., Minagi, S. et al. (1988). The aspect of dietary intake of full denture wearers. *J Jpn Prosthodont Soc*, 32, 774–779.

Scarmeas, N., Stern, Y., Tang, M.X. et al. (2006). Mediterranean diet and risk for Alzheimer's disease. *Ann Neurol*, 59(6), 912–921.

Shimizu, T., Ueda, T., & Sakurai, K. (2007). New method for evaluation of tongue-coating status. *J Oral Rehab*, 34(6), 442–447.

Sumi, Y., Ozawa, N., Michiwaki, Y. et al. (2012). Oral conditions and oral management approaches in mild dementia patients. *Nippon Ronen Igakkai Zasshi*, 49, 90–98.

Suzuki, H., Kanazawa, M., Komagamine, Y. et al. (2017). The effect of new complete denture fabrication and simplified dietary advice on nutrient intake and masticatory function of edentulous elderly: a randomized-controlled trial. *Clin Nutr*, 37(5), 1441–1447.

Tanaka, T., Hirano, H., Ohara, Y et al. (2021). Oral Frailty Index-8 in the risk assessment of new-onset oral frailty and functional disability among community-dwelling older adults. *Arch Gerontol Geriatr*, 94, 104340.

Tanaka, T., Takahashi, K., Hirano, H. et al. (2018). Oral frailty as a risk factor for physical frailty and mortality in community-dwelling elderly. *J Gerontol A Biol Sci Med Sci*, 73(12), 1661–1667.

United Nations (2015). Transforming our World: The 2030 Agenda for Sustainable Development, New York UN. https://sdgs.un.org/publications/transforming-our-world-2030-agenda-sustainable-development-17981 (accessed 30 June 2024).

Wakai, K., Naito, M., Naito, T. et al. (2010). Tooth loss and intake of nutrients and foods: A nationwide survey of Japanese dentists. *Community Dent Oral Epidemiol*, 38, 43–49.

World Health Organization (2015). *World Report on Ageing and Health*. Geneva: WHO. https://www.who.int/publications/i/item/9789241565042 (accessed 13 May 2024).

World Health Organization (2022). *Global Oral Health Status Report: Towards Universal Health Coverage for Oral Health by 2030*. Geneva: WHO. https://www.who.int/publications/i/item/9789240061484 (accessed 13 May 2024).

Yoneyama, T., Yoshida, M., Ohrui, T. et al. (2002). Oral Care Working Group. Oral care reduces pneumonia in older patients in nursing homes. *J Am Geriatr Soc*, 50(3), 430–433.

Yoshihara, A., Watanabe, R., Nishimuta, M et al. (2005). The relationship between dietary intake and the number of teeth in elderly Japanese subjects. *Gerodontology*, 22(4), 211–218. https://www.jda.or.jp/dentist/oral_frail/pdf/manual_all.pdf (accessed 13 May 2024).

3

The link between systemic health and oral health

Oral Health for an Ageing Population: Evidence, Policy, Practice and Evaluation, First Edition. Kakuhiro Fukai.
© 2025 John Wiley & Sons Ltd. Published 2025 by John Wiley & Sons Ltd.

3.1 Introduction

The maintenance of dental and oral health over a lifetime, as well as efforts to prevent tooth loss and retain and/or recover oral function, contributes to the prevention and control of non-communicable diseases (NCDs) (Botelho et al. 2022), which cause death or result in conditions requiring long-term care. Dental and oral health maintenance also help to slow the senescence (ageing) process and promote healthy and independent longevity by improving diet and social function. To what extent does the scientific evidence accumulated thus far support these claims? This chapter represents a wide-ranging, comprehensive review of the evidence regarding the effects of dental care and oral health on the various factors that damage health. This review leads us to a greater recognition, understanding and visualization of the relationship between oral health and whole-body health. The unambiguous conclusion is that we must reform our healthcare systems based on that recognition. An important step to achieving that is to propose new policies that promote interprofessional cooperation under the banner of 'health in all policies' (HiAP).

From a generational perspective, the current status of population ageing in Japan (where ageing has advanced the earliest and most quickly) can be described as follows: with the baby-boom generation (born during 1947–1949) turning 65 years old in 2012, the number of people aged 65 years and over reached 30.74 million, topping the 30-million mark for the first time ever. As a result, the percentage of the population aged 65 years and over has reached 24.1%, which breaks down to people aged 65–74 years accounting for 12.2% and those aged 75 years and over accounting for 11.9% [Ministry of Health, Labour and Welfare (MHLW) of Japan 2022].

Meanwhile, expenditures on social security benefits in Japan rose to JPY136.3 trillion in fiscal year 2020. Broken down by sector, this was JPY55.6 trillion for pension, JPY42.7 trillion for medical and dental care, and JPY11.4 trillion for long-term care (National Institute of Population and Social Security Research 2022). These numbers have been increasing continuously since the data were first published in 1950, calling into question the financial sustainability of maintaining a high-quality universal health insurance system that includes sufficient support for long-term care.

In order to overcome these formidable challenges, researchers and policymakers need to work together to create policies that strengthen and streamline the system in three general directions: (1) promoting cross-professional cooperation within and among the healthcare fields; (2) improving the availability and accessibility of evidence-based health information; and (3) implementing effective and sustainable measures for the prevention and control of NCDs and frailty, which often lead to dependency on long-term care and are the primary causes of death. Japan, which in 1961 established one of the world's first and longest-running universal health insurance systems, now faces the challenging task of improving and maintaining that system, with the ultimate aim being the realization of a society characterized by health, well-being and longevity.

These circumstances warrant a discussion about how the field of dental care and oral health can contribute to the realization of health and longevity. The goal of dental care and oral health is the lifelong maintenance of oral function, which more than two decades of accumulated evidence has shown to be closely linked to systemic health. However, because the fields of dentistry and medicine have developed separately in terms of education systems as well as funding, the obstacles to initiating and maintaining effective cooperation and collaboration are great. Evidence-based practice, however, exists as a common language and shared value of these two fields. The evidence on the contribution of oral health to general health leads to the conclusion that these two fields should move further towards uniting under the common HiAP banner.

This chapter aims to present a comprehensive overview and analysis of the current scientific evidence on the relationship between oral and general health, so that this evidence can be drawn upon when formulating policy recommendations. This evidence can also be used as the basis for discussing, planning and implementing future research programs and agendas.

3.2 Life expectancy and HLE

3.2.1 Determinants of average life expectancy and age-specific survival rates

Since the 1980s, Japan has been the world leader in longevity, with the average life expectancy among the Japanese reaching 81.6 years for men and 87.7 years for women in 2020 (MHLW of Japan 2022). Because the ageing phenomenon has been accompanied by a continuous downward trend in the birth rate, the result has been an overall ageing of the population structure, and the ageing of Japan is progressing at a speed that no other developed country has ever experienced. Moreover, the age-specific survival curves in 2020 reveal that the average expected remaining life span of 75-year-olds was 12.5 years for men and 16.2 years for women. Furthermore, the survival rates in that age group were 76.0% in men and 88.4% in women, and at age 90 the survival rates were 28.1% for men and 52.6% for women (MHLW of Japan 2022). The expected life span that must be taken into account from the perspective of healthcare, therefore, is much longer than the current average life span.

There is no doubt that human beings desire more than simple longevity. Rather, we want to live long lives that are also characterized by independence and well-being. Therefore, society must function in such a way that those of us living with disabilities have equal access to healthcare and support.

The rate of increase of average life expectancy in Japan has slowed somewhat since the 1980s (Ikeda et al. 2011). However, given that the maximum biological life span of humans is currently thought to be around 120 years (Fries 1980; Olshansky et al. 1990), it is likely that our life expectancy will continue to increase for the foreseeable future. At present, the percentage of people requiring long-term care is 2.8% for the 65–69 year age group, 5.5% for the 70–74 year age group, and 21.9% for those aged 75 years or older (MHLW of Japan 2020). Moreover, the average 'years of independence' (often referred to as an indicator of healthy longevity) has increased annually by 0.14 for men and 0.09 for women over the past 5 years (Seko et al. 2012; Hashimoto 2013). Although the ultimate goal is to prolong healthy life expectancy, if increasing average life expectancy is always accompanied by a proportional increase in healthy life expectancy, policies and practices designed to prolong average life expectancy actually do serve both purposes. In fact, a previous study has shown that while morbidity prevalence rates are on the rise due to population ageing across the world, disability rates are decreasing due to improved disease control measures (Ikeda et al. 2011).

As such, in order to make healthy longevity a reality, the following four goals should be given priority:

1) to increase life expectancy and prevent early death;
2) to prevent and delay dependence on long-term care;
3) To prevent a decline in living functions due to ageing;
4) to promote health throughout the life course.

Above all, enacting preventive measures against diseases that result in death and conditions leading to dependence on long-term care is an obvious priority. Approximately 70% of deaths in Japan are attributed to the main causes of death, such as cancer, heart disease, pneumonia and cerebrovascular disease (MHLW of Japan 2021). If these diseases were to be eliminated, an extension of life expectancy of 3–4 years can be expected in the case of cancer, 1.5 years in the case of heart disease, and 1 year in the case of pneumonia or cerebrovascular disease (MHLW of Japan 2021). Moreover, around 60% of long-term care dependency is caused by just three health conditions: cerebrovascular disease, dementia and falls/fractures (MHLW of Japan 2019). The prevention of these diseases, including joint disorders, will lead to an extension of the period of independent life.

Health promotion measures are effective in extending life expectancy. It is estimated that average life expectancy would increase by 1.8 years in men and 0.6 years in women if all adults quit smoking, and by 0.9 years in both men and women if systolic blood pressure among the Japanese population could be decreased to the level where adverse health effects are minimized (Ikeda et al. 2011). Moreover, to further enhance population health, it is necessary to tackle other risk factors such as hyperglycaemia, lack of exercise, alcohol consumption, excessive weight and obesity, and high salt intake, in addition to smoking and high blood pressure (Ikeda et al. 2011).

The factors that damage health are genetic, lifestyle-related, healthcare system-related, and social determinants. Among these, the genetic factor accounts for 25–30% of health problems that lead to death (Schroeder 2007; Christensen et al. 2009). Lifestyle and social environment factors account for a larger percentage than genetic background, a fact that needs to be taken into consideration when judging disease risk (Robertson et al. 1977; Takeya et al. 1984). Many of the risk factors for healthy longevity, most of which are NCDs, are also risk factors for dental and oral health. These are called 'common risk factors'.

3.2.2 Ageing and daily living functions

This section deals with ageing, which is a topic that cannot be avoided when discussing life span extension. Apart from diseases, causes of death include ageing and accidents. For whatever reason, when cells and organs that consist of groups of cells (tissues) can no longer function, humans become incapable of maintaining the functions necessary for survival as an individual organism, and this results in death. Moreover, the process leading to death varies depending on the condition or disease that causes the decline in organ function. Before it finally leads to death, ageing usually results in a period of restricted activities of daily living (ADLs), meaning that a person is unable to live independently. This period of activity restriction may extend over a long period of time in some cases, such as with dementia, while cancer and other diseases often cause a relatively short period of dependence (Lynn 2011).

Ageing can be defined as the changes one experiences due to a gradually progressing decline in physical functions that occurs as one ages. Ageing at the organ level can be attributed to damage to the types of cells that have little or no ability to divide, such as brain, nerve and myocardial cells. For most other types of cells, ageing occurs when cells stop dividing after completing approximately 50 cycles of division (Hayflick et al. 1961). Thus, all organs age as one gets older, and the ageing of organs manifests in the form of reduced functionality. This cannot be avoided in humans.

Despite this decline in organ function due to ageing, all organs function together in a complementary manner to maintain an overall physical condition that allows everyday life to be carried out without significant difficulty. However, a variety of factors gradually lead to various physical and psychological symptoms and conditions that are commonly observed in older people, and which are collectively referred to as geriatric syndromes (Sasaki 2008). This often leads to a decrease in ADLs, after which complete recovery is unlikely, meaning that long-term care and rehabilitation based on multidisciplinary collaboration within a community, in addition to medical treatment, come to play an increasingly important role.

The oral cavity is also an organ, so the risk factors involved in mouth ageing must be researched and assessed just like any other organ. Such research seeks to identify the extent to which the decline of oral status and various oral functions (e.g. number of teeth, saliva flow, tongue pressure, bite force) contribute to the overall ageing of the mouth. For example, the number of remaining teeth, which are necessary for the daily feeding function, decreases with age (Fukai et al. 2011). As the various oral functions begin to decline, the mouth experiences frailty just like the body does – thus the increasing prevalence of the term 'oral frailty'. This affects food intake, so the extent to which the progress of overall body ageing can be slowed by maintaining dental and oral health is another area that requires further investigation.

3.3   Scientific evidence and health policy

Proposed in 1991 by Gordon Guyatt at McMaster University in Canada and followed by an article in the American medical journal *JAMA* a year later, the concept of evidence-based medicine (EBM) quickly took hold as a revolutionary movement that changed the medical field in significant and irreversible ways (Evidence-Based Medicine Working Group 1992). Thirty years have elapsed since then, and the evidence-based approach is today widely adopted in health policy as well (Gray 1997).

This approach represents a playbook that can be followed to establish a scientific basis for decision-making among concerned parties in clinical and policymaking settings. At the same time, they serve to ensure the quality and reliability of the health information available to all stakeholders. The amount of health information has grown to such an extent that opinions and assumptions based on individual experiences are no longer considered to be sufficient grounds for establishing or continuing practices that impact people's health. The vastly improved availability and access to large amounts of evidence-based information allows health policymakers to utilize limited resources more efficiently.

Evidence is obtained by analysing and synthesizing the results of previous studies, and there are several levels of evidence (Aihara et al. 2010; Fukui et al. 2014). The levels of evidence are determined by the type of outcome factor and the study design. The level of evidence also depends on whether the aim is to observe facts and find correlations, to demonstrate a causal relationship based on the results of a follow-up or intervention, or to statistically verify the results of several studies. Based on the level of evidence, study designs can be broadly classified into (in order of increasing strength of the evidence generated): (1) observational studies, (2) intervention studies, and (3) data integration studies.

Observational studies include case reports, cross-sectional studies and cohort studies. Intervention studies can be non-randomized or randomized controlled studies, depending on whether participant allocation is determined randomly. Data integration studies include systematic reviews, in which existing study results are systematically analysed, and meta-analyses, in which comparable data are collected from several studies and statistically combined to arrive at an overall conclusion that is more strongly evidence-based.

In the clinical setting, EBM is employed to draw up clinical guidelines, which are in turn utilized to determine the proper treatment for each patient. In this case, the starting point is to set a clinical question. This is normally done via the PICO (or PECO) format, which involves making decisions about who the subjects are (P: patient, population, problem), what treatment is likely to be effective (I or E: intervention, indicator, exposure), what the treatment should be compared with (C: comparison, control), and what possible outcomes are expected (O: outcome) (Fukui et al. 2007). Basically, the same methods and procedures can be used in evidence-based health policy (EBHP) – it simply requires changing 'clinicians' to 'policymakers' and 'treatment' to 'health policy'. In addition, evidence is integral to both the process and evaluation of policy making, and evidence is also fundamental to both understanding and improving practice (Boaz et al. 2019).

3.4 Evidence linking dental care and oral health to prolonged HLE

3.4.1 Conceptual pathway of oral health and HLE

An accumulation of evidence has established a strong relationship between oral and general health, and there are two general pathways whereby dental care and oral health contribute to healthy longevity: (1) health promotion activities, and (2) reduction in the risk of disease. The first pathway involves promotion of healthy behaviour such as exercise, nutrition and rest. The second pathway involves reducing risk factors for NCDs and preventing the onset and worsening of diseases that lead to death or dependency on long-term care.

Based on the results of previous research, Figure 3.1 presents a conceptual pathway detailing how the maintenance of dental and oral health and the maintenance and recovery of oral functions through dental care can contribute to HLE, which is defined as the maintenance of quality of life (QOL), ADLs and extension of life expectancy (Fukai 2013). This visual conceptual pathway is useful for providing a simple and easily understandable explanation to policymakers, the media and the general population.

In the following sections, the evidence for each component of this pathway is presented in turn.

3.4.2 The association of tooth loss and chewing function with life expectancy

First, we will look at the relationship between dental/oral health status and life expectancy. Number of teeth is a strong indicator of oral health. There is also a great deal of evidence linking number of teeth to general health, including life expectancy (Shimazaki et al. 2001; Abnet et al. 2005; Fukai et al. 2007; Osterberg et al. 2008; Ansai et al. 2010; Peng et al. 2019; Beukers et al. 2021).

One of the most significant of these studies, a cohort study showing that prevention of tooth loss contributes to prolongation of life expectancy, was conducted by my own research group. This was a 15-year cohort study of 5730 local residents between the ages of 40 and 89, and it found a clear association between tooth retention at baseline and survival prognosis.

This study is still ongoing, having reached the 30-year point as I write, and the results have become even stronger and clearer. At the 15-year point, the cumulative survival rate of men in the age range of

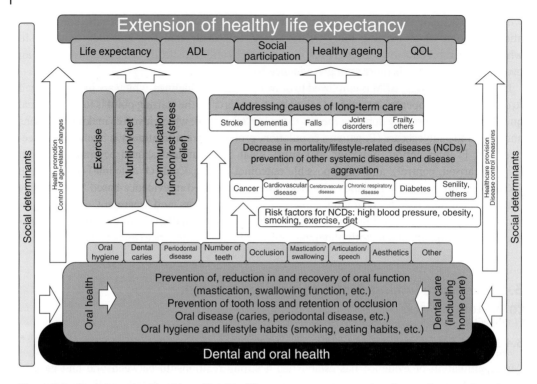

Figure 3.1 Dental care/oral health and healthy life expectancy: conceptual pathways. *Source:* Adapted from Fukai et al. (2013).

80–89 years who had 10 or more functional teeth was twice as high as those with fewer than 10 teeth, and the mean survival time was extended by about 2.5 years. In women in the same age group, the survival rate was about 1.5 times higher in those with more remaining teeth. When confounding factors such as systemic disease were adjusted for all participants over the age of 40, the relationship between the number of teeth and life expectancy was stronger in men than in women, with a hazard ratio (HR) of 1.33 [95% confidence interval (CI): 1.11–1.59, $P = 0.01$] (Fukai et al. 2007) (Figure 3.2). The reason for this is that men have a shorter life expectancy. Regarding the assessment of the critical tooth number (CTN) required for prevention of subjective dysphagia caused by oral impairments and the evaluation of the relationship between this CTN and mortality, our results were as follows. The average functional tooth number of participants with and without subjective dysphagia declined with age in both sexes. The CTNs for each age group (40s, 50s, 60s, 70s and 80s) not including the denture group were 20.0, 17.5, 14.0, 11.8 and 10.1 in men and 19.0, 14.7, 12.7, 9.5 and 4.0 in women, respectively. These CTNs were significant factors of 15-year mortality in both sexes ($P < 0.05$). The HRs were 0.72 (95% CI: 0.55–0.93) in men and 0.71 (0.51–0.99) in women. In older people, the minimum number of functional teeth needed to avoid subjective dysphagia might not be as high as in young people (Fukai et al 2008) (Figure 3.3).

Another study investigated the relationship between average life expectancy and the average number of remaining teeth in the Japanese population over the past 30 years, finding a correlation coefficient of 0.96 in men and 0.92 in women and establishing a clear and significant linear relationship (Fukai et al. 2010). A higher number of remaining teeth indicates better oral functions, which has clearly contributed to the prolongation of the life expectancy of the Japanese population.

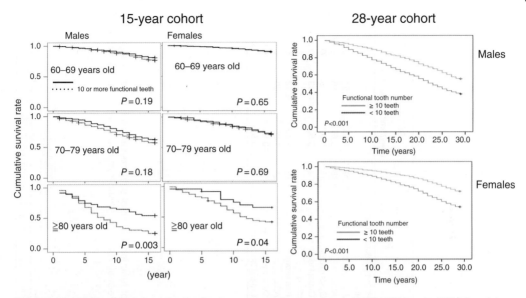

Figure 3.2 Number of teeth and mortality. Long-term cohort study: *n* = 5742 (2256 male, 3486 female) community residents over 40 years old. *Sources:* Fukai et al. (2007, 2018).

Many other studies have added to the robust body of evidence establishing a link between tooth loss and morality. These are described in the following paragraphs: In a 6-year cohort study of 929 Japanese institutionalized older people (mean age 80 years) conducted by Shimazaki et al. (2001), mortality was found to be 1.8 times higher in participants with no teeth (and no dentures) than in those with 20 or more teeth [odds ratio (OR): 1.8, 95% CI: 1.1–2.8] (Shimazaki et al. 2001).

In a 15-year cohort study of 28 790 Chinese community residents in the age range of 40–69 by Abnet et al. (2005), mortality was 1.1 times higher in participants with a tooth loss rate higher than the median for their age, relative to those below the median HR (1.13, 95% CI: 1.09–1.18) (Abnet et al. 2005).

In a 24-year cohort study by Cabrera et al. (2005) in Sweden consisting of 1462 female community residents between the ages of 38 and 60, mortality was 1.3 times higher in participants with 11 or more missing teeth compared with those with 10 or fewer missing teeth (HR = 1.27, 95% CI: 1.09–1.47) (Cabrera et al. 2005).

In a 10-year cohort study by Morita et al. (2006) of 118 institutionalized elderly Japanese (80 years and older), mortality was 2.7 times higher in men with fewer than 20 teeth compared with those with 20 or more teeth (HR = 2.71, 95% CI: 1.05–7.05) (Morita et al. 2006).

In a 15-year cohort study by Fukai et al. (2007) which consisted of 5830 Japanese community residents between the ages of 40 and 89, mortality was 1.3 times higher in men with fewer than 10 teeth, relative to those with 10 or more functional teeth (HR = 1.33, 95% CI: 1.11–1.59) (Fukai et al. 2007).

In a 15.5-year cohort study by Padilha et al. (2008) in the United States consisting of 500 community residents with a mean age of 57, mortality in the group with 1–19 teeth was 2.2 times higher than that of the group with 20 or more teeth (HR = 2.17, 95% CI: 1.50–3.13), and the group with no teeth had a mortality rate 1.8 times higher than the group with 20 or more teeth (HR = 1.76, 95% CI: 1.04–2.98).

In a 21-year cohort study by Holm-Pedersen et al. (2008) in Denmark consisting of 573 institutionalized individuals between the ages 70 and 90, mortality was 1.3 times higher in those with no teeth than in those with 20 or more teeth (HR = 1.26, 95% CI: 1.03–1.55).

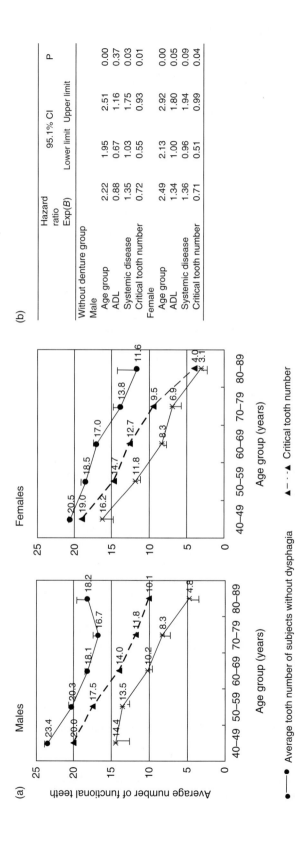

Figure 3.3 Critical number of functional teeth without dysphagia and mortality. (a) Average number of functional teeth of subjects with/without dysphagia and critical tooth number at each age group for subjects without dentures. (b) Survivals of male/female subjects by age group, systemic disease and number of functional teeth in Cox regression model. *Source:* Fukai et al. 2011 / John Wiley & Sons.

In a 12-year cohort study by Holmlund et al. (2010) in Sweden consisting of 7674 participants (including both institutionalized and community residents) between the ages of 20 and 89, mortality was 1.6 times higher (HR = 1.56, 95% CI: 1.15–2.13) in the group with 20–25 teeth than in the group with 26 or more teeth. HRs for groups with 15–19 teeth, 10–14 teeth, and fewer than 10 teeth were 2.33 (95% CI: 1.66–3.27), 2.11 (95% CI: 1.44–3.10) and 2.75 (95% CI: 1.81–4.16), respectively (Holmlund et al. 2010).

In a 4-year cohort study by Hayasaka et al. (2013) consisting of 21 730 Japanese community residents 65 years of age or older, mortality in participants with 10–19 teeth (no dentures) was 1.3 times higher (HR = 1.34, 95% CI: 1.09–1.64) and mortality of those with 0–9 teeth (no dentures) was 1.7 times higher (HR = 1.73, 95% CI: 1.47–2.04) than in those with 20 or more teeth (Hayasaka et al. 2013).

In a study by Ando et al. (2014) of 7779 male community residents between ages 40 and 79, mortality among participants between ages 40 and 64 was 1.9 times higher (HR = 1.94, 95% CI: 1.09–3.43) in those with 10-19 teeth and 2.8 times higher (HR = 2.75, 95% CI: 1.37–5.49) in the group with no teeth, relative to those with 20 or more teeth.

The association of tooth loss with mortality from all causes, cardiovascular disease, coronary heart disease and cancer has been established for many years (Peng et al. 2019; Ishikawa et al. 2020; Maekawa et al, 2020; Beukers et al. 2021; Kotronia et al. 2021).

With regard to the effect of masticatory function and occlusal status on life expectancy, individuals with high masticatory function and people with occlusal stability (i.e. able to chew in the molar regions) have better health status and significantly lower mortality risk (Shimazaki et al. 2001; Schwahn et al. 2013). An association between masticatory function and cardiovascular disease mortality has also been reported (Aida et al. 2011).

Moreover, a subjective indicator of oral function assessment, i.e. whether or not one 'can chew anything', has been shown to be associated with the subsequent vital prognosis in male community residents in adulthood and later life (HR = 1.31, 95% CI: 1.07–1.6, $P = 0.01$) (Fukai et al. 2011). The complaint, 'I cannot chew well' was associated with increased mortality rate. Chewing ability is associated with mortality of older adults and may be a predictor of survival rate (Ansai et al. 2007).

3.4.3 Oral health and the leading causes of death

In terms of the relationship between oral health and diseases that are among the leading causes of death, some reports suggest that number of teeth is related to death due to heart and respiratory diseases (Fukai et al. 2007; Aida et al. 2011; Kotronia et al. 2021). Moreover, many reports suggest a relationship between periodontal disease and NCDs (Khader et al. 2006; Tonetti et al. 2007; Demmer et al. 2010; Teeuw et al. 2010; Demmer et al. 2012; Janket et al. 2015; Botelho et al. 2022).

Periodontal disease is no longer seen as merely a local intraoral infection, but rather as a sustained chronic inflammatory disease. Therefore, the idea that periodontal disease affects systemic diseases is becoming more commonly accepted, as is the possibility that periodontal disease may serve as a progression-promoting factor for diabetes mellitus and arterial stiffening.

For example, Morita et al. (2010) reported that in a 4-year cohort study of 1023 adults, an association was found between periodontal pockets (CPI 3 or more) and the development of metabolic syndrome conditions such as obesity, hypertension and dyslipidaemia (OR = 1.6, 95% CI: 1.1–2.2).

In this section, I review the association of dental and oral health with leading causes of death and NCDs, finding evidence of associations between dental and oral health and diabetes mellitus, cardiovascular diseases, cancer, respiratory diseases and metabolic syndrome.

3.4.3.1 Diabetes mellitus

Diabetes mellitus has been established as a risk factor for diseases in the oral cavity, and periodontal disease in particular is closely associated with diabetes mellitus. For this reason, dentists have a potential role in contributing to the prevention of the incidence and worsening of diabetes mellitus. Moreover, as performing oral health management can potentially result in early detection of diabetes mellitus and provide opportunities to educate patients in the pre-diabetic stage, medical–dental cooperation should be further promoted in this area.

In Japan, medical clinical guidelines for the treatment of diabetes include periodontal disease as a risk factor, while dental clinical guidelines for the treatment of periodontal disease include diabetes as a risk factor. It is quite rare for medical clinical guidelines to include such specific dental-related information. This illustrates just how well-accepted the association between periodontitis and diabetes is in both the medical and dental communities. The medical clinical guidelines (Japanese Society for Diabetes 2019) are as follows:

- What is periodontal disease?
  - Periodontal disease is an inflammatory disease involving plaque bacteria and is broadly classified into gingivitis, in which inflammation is confined to the gingiva, and periodontitis, which involves a loss of supporting tissue.
  - Periodontal disease is a disease of the oral cavity that is reported to affect approximately 80% of Japanese individuals of middle age or older, and it is the foremost cause of dental extraction.
  - The treatment of periodontal disease entails not only establishing plaque control in affected patients, but also reducing inflammation through plaque and calculus removal from periodontal pockets and ensuring routine post-removal periodontal maintenance care aimed at preventing a relapse of the disease (Araki et al. 2020).
- Does diabetes influence the onset/progression of periodontal disease?
  - Periodontal disease has been shown to occur more frequently among patients with type 1 diabetes in comparison to young, healthy individuals (Takahashi et al. 2001).
  - The risk of the onset of periodontal disease and the progression of alveolar bone resorption is significantly increased in patients with type 2 diabetes and an HbA1c value of $\geq 6.5\%$ (Morita et al. 2012).
- Is diabetes treatment effective in improving periodontal disease?
  - Diabetes treatment may lead to the improvement of periodontal tissue inflammation (Katagiri et al. 2013).
- Does periodontal disease affect glycaemic control?
  - Periodontal disease as an inflammatory disease has been epidemiologically shown to adversely affect glycaemic control (Demmer et al. 2008).
  - As periodontal disease becomes more severe, it becomes more difficult to achieve glycaemic control in affected patients (Graziani et al. 2018).
- Is treating periodontal disease effective in improving glycaemic control?
  - The treatment of periodontal disease has been shown to lead to improvement in the glycaemic status of some patients with type 2 diabetes (Engebretson et al. 2013; Simpson et al. 2015).

3.4.3.2 Cardiovascular disease

An association between periodontal and cardiovascular diseases has been observed. Recent studies have found that the risk of cardiovascular disease for people aged 65 years or younger is higher among those with periodontal disease, that the association of periodontal disease with acute myocardial infarction is stronger than with chronic coronary heart disease, and that people with periodontal disease accompanied by systemic bacterial infection have a higher risk of coronary heart disease. A few studies have revealed that treating periodontal disease is associated with a reduced risk of developing cardiovascular disease and a decrease in serum antibody titres, but these have not yet been established as causal relationships (Fukai et al. 2009; Chen et al. 2012; Watt et al. 2012; Liljestrand, et al. 2015; Dietrich et al. 2017; Lee et al. 2019; Sanz et al 2020; Gao et al. 2021; Blaschke et al. 2022).

3.4.3.3 Cancer

One of the risk factors for cancer is dietary intake and nutrition. Evidence regarding the association between dental/oral health and diet/nutrition are presented and discussed later in this chapter.

In addition to the common risk factors of dental/oral health and cancer (such as smoking, diet and obesity), there is also evidence that dental/oral healthcare and management can improve the outcome of cancer-related surgery. For example, the link between cancer and oral health is seen in the fact that oral adverse events (such as stomatitis) that occur due to cancer treatment can hinder treatment and affect patients' vital prognosis. Some evidence suggests that the implementation of proper oral hygiene management before initiating cancer treatment is effective in decreasing the risk of these oral adverse events and reducing their severity (Otake et al. 2022).

There are some reports which show the association between cancer and oral diseases/number of teeth (Hiraki et al. 2008; Wang et al. 2013; Chen et al. 2015; Nwizu et al. 2020; Gao et al. 2021; Guo et al. 2021; Albuquerque-Souza and Sahingur 2022; Kesharani et al. 2022; Amato 2023).

A 2018 study by Shi et al. (2017) has provided the strongest evidence to date that tooth loss is associated with cancer incidence. This was a dose–response meta-analysis of over 30 000 cases from 11 countries, and it found that cancer risk increases by 9% for every 10 teeth lost. This association was even stronger for types of cancer that occur near the oral cavity, such as head and neck, lung and oesophageal. The authors propose a number of possible pathways to explain the relationship between tooth loss and cancer, such as chronic systemic inflammation, carbohydrate intake and oral microbial accumulation. This last point receives additional support from Albuquerque-Souza and Sahingur (2022), who propose a connection between periodontitis, gut microbiota and immunity.

3.4.3.4 Chronic obstructive pulmonary disease and respiratory disease

Pneumonia is a major cause of mortality and morbidity among older adults worldwide. Community-acquired pneumonia (CAP) is a leading cause of morbidity among community-dwelling older adults in many countries and is different from hospital-acquired pneumonia and ventilator-associated pneumonia. The overall incidence rates (per 100 000 older adults, $\geq$ 65 years) of CAP have been estimated as 1790–4000 in Japan (2015); 630–1463 in the US (2015), and 1400 in Europe (2013). A recent report showed that 6.8 million cases of clinical pneumonia, including CAP, resulted in hospital admissions of older adults globally (Iwai-Saito et al. 2021).

A 2-year cohort study of elderly nursing home residents by Yoneyama et al. (2002) found that regular oral care yielded a 40% reduction in the incidence of pneumonia. The idea that oral care can help to prevent aspiration pneumonia in elderly patients has already become widely accepted; however, this claim rests primarily on evidence from this single randomized controlled trial (RCT), so further accumulation of evidence from well-planned RCTs is needed.

Sufficient evidence also exists to support a connection between oral care and the prevention of ventilator-associated pneumonia. An investigation into whether and how oral care improves the outcome of cancer surgery was conducted with mortality and incidence of pneumonia as the outcome variables (Ishimaru et al. 2018). The data source was the national medical information database maintained by the Japanese MHLW. The participants in this study were approximately 510 000 patients who underwent tumour resection or tumorectomy of the head and neck, oesophagus, stomach, colon cancer, lung or liver. The data analysis indicated that 3.3% of patients who received preoperative oral care by a dentist contracted postoperative pneumonia, compared with 3.8% of those who did not receive oral care, a 13.2% reduction. Especially, oral hygiene reduces the mortality from aspiration pneumonia in frail older adults (Müller 2015). In addition, Takeuchi et al. (2019) reported that periodontitis is associated with chronic obstructive pulmonary disease.

3.4.3.5 Risk factors of metabolic syndrome and other NCDs

Among reports from various countries regarding the association between metabolic syndrome and oral health, there have been a relatively large number of studies conducted in Japan. Individuals with metabolic syndrome have a high risk of periodontal disease, and some studies have shown that metabolic syndrome is more prevalent among those with periodontal disease; however, the majority of this evidence is from cross-sectional studies. Obesity, which plays a central role in metabolic syndrome, is an important risk factor for diabetes mellitus and arteriosclerotic diseases. Many studies have shown that obesity is also associated with periodontal disease, and in particular, a strong association has been found between visceral fat obesity and periodontitis. As many aspects of the relationship between metabolic syndrome and oral health, such as the directionality and underlying mechanisms of the association, remain unclear, more evidence needs to be accumulated in order to further understand this association (Nascimento et al. 2016; Machado et al. 2020; Botelho et al. 2022; Zhao et al. 2022).

With respect to NCD risk factors, smoking, drinking, exercise, and eating habits have each been found to be associated with oral health problems such as periodontal disease. In particular, smoking clearly affects periodontal health. Although it has been suggested that intake of a large amount of alcohol may affect periodontal health, results have varied among studies (Sheihamu and Watt 2000; Hanioka et al. 2011; Watt and Sheiham 2012; Botelho et al. 2022).

People with good exercise habits and those who consume healthy food and nutrients tend to have better periodontal health. Improved lifestyle habits bring about positive effects not only for systemic health but also for oral health, but further evidence is required to justify the inclusion of instruction regarding lifestyle habits (other than smoking) in oral health guidance programmes and routines.

3.4.4 Oral health and the leading causes of long-term care dependence

3.4.4.1 Oral health and long-term care dependence

When a person becomes dependent on long-term care, their ADLs are restricted, so it should be no surprise that their oral health condition will decline. Indeed, a number of studies have shown this to be true. On the other hand, there is also evidence indicating that worsening oral health condition predicts future onset of conditions leading to long-term care dependence, as well as a general decline in physical functions (Furuta et al. 2013).

Predictive factors for the incidence of conditions that lead to long-term care dependence include old age, cognitive dysfunction, visual impairment, low subjective health, decreased or increased body mass index, decreased functionality in the extremities, decreased exercise or social interaction, and smoking (Fujinami et al. 2021; Iwasaki et al. 2021).

It has been observed that oral health may be related to some of these predictive factors. For example, oral health affects social activities, such as interacting with friends and participating in recreational activities, because it affects conversational ability, facial appearance and smile, and eating function (Fukai et al. 2022). For the elderly, social participation has been shown to have a preventive effect on the development and progression of conditions that lead to long-term care dependence, and thus it is likely that oral health status plays an important role in delaying long-term care dependence via its effect on social participation.

Among elderly people with few remaining teeth, a clear association between denture use and longevity has been reported (Fukai et al. 2008). It is therefore likely that increased dissemination of healthcare interventions aimed at maintaining or improving oral function, such as implants and dentures, can reduce the incidence of dependence on long-term care. However, more evidence is needed to strengthen this claim.

Aida et al. (2012) conducted a 4-year cohort study of community residents aged 65 and over, and found that elderly people with 19 teeth or fewer had a 1.21-fold higher risk of becoming dependent on long-term care than those with 20 teeth or more, and this difference was significant.

Dementia and falls are among the top causes of dependence on long-term care. Yamamoto et al. (2012a) conducted a 4-year cohort study of 4425 community residents, reporting that the incidence of dementia was 1.85-fold (95% CI: 1.04–3.31) higher in people with 19 teeth or fewer and no dentures, compared with those with 20 teeth or more.

With regard to the relationship between tooth retention and physical symptoms, I co-authored a study of local residents aged 40 years old or more and found a correlation between tooth loss and 10 symptoms, including pain in the lower back, shoulders, upper limbs and lower limbs. Dividing the participants into three groups based on the number of functional teeth (0–9, 10–19 and 20+), we found that, for both men and women, the groups with fewer functional teeth had more of these symptoms (Fukai et al. 2009).

Oral health status has also been shown to be associated with the prevention of long-term care dependence. A 4-year follow-up study of 4000 community residents over the age of 65 found that those with limited masticatory function had a risk of long-term care dependence that was 1.3 times greater than those with no masticatory limitation (Aida et al. 2012).

3.4.4.2 Frailty and oral health

Frailty is highly prevalent in old age and confers high risk for falls, disability, hospitalization and mortality. The 'frailty cycle' proposed by Fried is a vicious circle model involving decreasing muscle strength and mass (sarcopenia), fatigue and decreasing energy consumption. The model demonstrates that nutritional factors such as loss of appetite, weight loss and low nutrition are accelerators of frailty (Fried et al. 2001; Xue 2011). Oral health is closely related to low nutrition and muscle mass (Iwasaki et al. 2021; Tanaka et al. 2021).

Poor oral health is common among older adults and can impair essential ADLs and contribute to frailty (Minakuchi et al. 2016; Watanabe et al. 2017; Tanaka et al. 2018; Shirobe et al. 2021).

In a 4-year follow-up study of 2000 community residents, those with low nutrition caused by reduced oral function were 2.4 times more likely to be diagnosed with physical frailty and had 2.2 times greater risk of mortality (Tanaka et al. 2018).

Researchers are now recommending that oral health indicators be added to the operational definition of frailty. The new definition would include age-related loss of oral function as a factor in malnutrition, which in turn affects cognitive and physical functional decline (Dibello et al. 2021, 2023; Matsubara et al. 2021; Nagatani et al. 2023).

3.4.4.3 Cerebrovascular disease and oral health

The disease that most frequently results in long-term care among the Japanese population is cerebrovascular disease. Cerebrovascular disease causes movement disorders that affect not only the extremities but also the orofacial area, and it can also cause the deterioration of oral hygienic status. Investigations of the association between oral health status and cerebrovascular diseases have revealed that young people and people with many missing teeth or high clinical attachment loss and periodontal probing depth (PPD) have an increased risk of stroke (Sen et al. 2018; Cardoso et al. 2023).

Moreover, periodontal disease has a stronger association with non-haemorrhagic (ischaemic) stroke than with haemorrhagic stroke. However, the current evidence on the association between periodontal disease maintenance risk of cerebrovascular events is insufficient to establish causality. It is necessary to conduct follow-up and/or intervention studies in order to address these issues (Janket et al. 2003; Khader et al. 2004; Sfyroeras et al. 2012; Sen and Mascari 2020; Mascari et al. 2021).

3.4.4.4 Falls and joint disease, and oral health

The question of whether poor oral status increases the risk of future incidence of falls and femoral neck fracture, as well as which oral conditions are associated with falls and fractures, has been investigated. Several cohort studies have demonstrated that loss of occlusal support and non-use of dentures after tooth loss are risk factors for subsequent fall events (Yamamoto and Naito 2015). Moreover, having periodontal disease and fewer teeth has been shown to increase the risk of subsequent femoral neck fracture.

In another, similar, 3-year cohort study of 1765 participants aged 65 years old and older, people with fewer teeth and no dentures had a 2.5-fold higher risk of falls (95% CI: 1.21–5.17) (Yamamoto et al. 2012b).

The relationship between oral health and joint diseases has been investigated via intervention studies, case-control studies, cross-sectional studies, and basic studies. The results suggest an association between periodontal disease and rheumatoid arthritis, and that the prevention and treatment of periodontal disease could improve some of the symptoms of rheumatoid arthritis (Hanada and Nomura 2015). However, these improvements were limited, and the degree of improvement is ambiguous in some of the articles; therefore, further investigative research is necessary.

3.4.4.5 Dementia and oral health

The question of whether oral health is associated with the subsequent onset of dementia or cognitive decline has been investigated in original articles reporting on cross-sectional and intervention studies. The majority of such studies have reported significant associations (Fang et al. 2018). Oral hygiene, periodontal disease, number of teeth, occlusion, mastication, dental visitation and whether an individual has a regular primary care dental clinic have all been reported as factors that are likely to be associated with the onset of dementia and cognitive decline.

3.4.4.5.1 Oral health behaviour and oral health care and dementia   Two cohort studies have examined the link between oral health behaviour and subsequent onset of dementia. In the first, the HR for dementia of those responding that they did not engage in daily oral hygiene behaviours was 1.76 (95% CI: 0.96–3.20), that of those who said they could not chew well was 1.47 (95% CI: 0.95–2.25), and that of those who indicated that they did not have a regular dental clinic was 1.44 (95% CI: 1.04–2.01) (Yamamoto et al. 2012a). In the second study, women who brushed their teeth less than three times a day had an HR for dementia of 1.65 (95% CI: 1.05–2.62), while women who visited dental clinics less than twice a year had an HR of 1.89 (95% CI: 1.21–2.95) (Paganini-Hill et al. 2012).

Two intervention studies on the relationship between oral care provided by caregivers and cognitive decline have been reported, and both showed that those who received oral care experienced a significant reduction in cognitive decline as measured by the Mini Mental State Examination (MMSE) (Kikutani et al. 2010).

In addition, there have been two case–control studies (Kimura and Kanzaki 2014; Gil-Montoya et al. 2017) investigating the relationship of oral care status and cognitive decline assessed by the MMSE. In the first, significant differences were observed between the good oral care and poor oral care groups (Kimura and Kanzaki 2014), and the second showed a significant association between the degree of cognitive impairment and oral hygiene status as operationalized by plaque accumulation and gingival bleeding (Gil-Montoya et al. 2017).

Taken together, these studies provide a strong indication that regular and continuous dental intervention is likely to be effective in preventing the onset of, and an increase in the severity of, cognitive decline. However, the strength of this claim is limited due to the low number of studies and the lack of a meta-analysis to date. Regular dental care also provides benefits for people experiencing cognitive decline that go beyond cognitive function, such as opportunities for social interaction.

3.4.4.5.2 *Nutrition and dementia* Epidemiological findings reported since 2000 show that diet and nutrition can have a mitigating effect on the onset of Alzheimer's disease (Barberger-Gateau et al. 2002; Morris et al. 2003). A low-calorie diet reduces oxidative stress, thereby providing a protective effect against cognitive decline (Mattson et al. 2002), and a high-calorie diet can lead to increased oxidative stress and is therefore considered to be a risk factor for cognitive impairment (Butterfield et al. 2002). In addition, a number of reports have found evidence that the Mediterranean diet (olive oil, whole grains, vegetables, nuts, etc.) acts prophylactically on cognitive decline (Scarmeas et al. 2006; Lourida et al. 2013; Shah 2013; Singh et al. 2014; Trichopoulou et al. 2015).

In addition, a cohort study conducted by Ozawa et al. (2013) (the Hisayama-cho Study) revealed that a diet including large amounts of soybeans and soybean products, green and yellow vegetables, light-coloured vegetables, algae, milk and other dairy products, and low rice intake is associated with a significantly lower risk of developing dementia.

In a cohort study conducted in 2014 in Japan, a significant negative association was observed between higher intake of milk and other dairy products and the incidence of dementia (diagnosed by DSM-III-R), Alzheimer's disease, and cerebrovascular dementia (Ozawa et al. 2014). Dairy intake may therefore work prophylactically against cognitive decline.

In addition, in a 2015 intervention study, intentional weight loss due to dietary restrictions was found to be associated with cognitive improvement in those with mild cognitive impairment (MCI) (Horie et al. 2016), and another study found that nutritional education programmes for caregivers of Alzheimer's disease patients had a positive effect on the cognitive function of patients (Rivière et al. 2001). These studies indicate that providing dietary guidance to the families and caregivers of the elderly is also effective in preventing cognitive decline.

In developed countries, the frequency of dental visitation is higher than that of medical checkups and treatment. In Japan, for example, half of the population reports having visited a dentist in the past year (Japan Dental Association 2016), and most people have easy access to dental care. Therefore, providing dietary guidance in dental clinics has great potential as a powerful public health approach to reducing cognitive decline among the population at large. For this reason, dental clinics should make heightened efforts to develop and enhance their dietary instruction content and procedures.

3.4.4.5.3 Relationship between cognitive decline and periodontal disease Ten cohort studies (Kaye et al. 2010; Arrivé et al. 2013; Batty et al. 2013; Naorungroj et al. 2013, 2015; Ide et al. 2016; Iwasaki et al. 2016; Tzeng et al. 2016; Chen et al. 2017; Lee et al. 2017b) and three case–control studies (Noble et al. 2014; Cestari et al. 2016; Lee et al. 2017a) have examined the association between periodontal status and subsequent cognitive decline or onset of dementia, with both significant and non-significant results. One cohort study (Arrivé et al. 2013) with onset of dementia as the outcome showed no significant association, but three case–control studies (Noble et al. 2014; Cestari et al. 2016; Lee et al. 2017a) showed significant association. There have been six reports with cognitive decline as the outcome (Kaye et al. 2010; Batty et al. 2013; Naorungroj et al. 2013, 2015; Ide et al. 2016; Iwasaki et al. 2016), three of which were significant (Kaye et al. 2010; Iwasaki et al. 2016; Ide et al. 2016), with the remaining three reports (Batty et al. 2013; Naorungroj et al. 2013, 2015) showing no significance.

However, if only studies conducted since 2015 are included, almost every study with dementia as the outcome has found significant associations (Naorungroj et al. 2015; Cestari et al. 2016; Ide et al. 2016; Iwasaki et al. 2016; Tzeng et al. 2016; Chen et al. 2017; Lee et al. 2017a, 2017b). One review in 2017 found that severe periodontal disease and Alzheimer's disease were significantly related (Leira et al. 2017). From these, it is clear that the claim that the prevention of periodontal disease contributes to delaying the onset of dementia is warranted.

In addition, given that periodontal disease is also a major cause of tooth loss, there are probably two pathways by which oral health prevention contributes to the prevention and delay of cognitive decline. The first a direct path, whereby periodontal disease prevention itself delays/prevents the onset of cognitive decline and dementia, and the second is an indirect path, whereby periodontal disease prevention activities prevent tooth loss, which in turn delays/prevents cognitive decline.

3.4.4.5.4 Relationship between tooth loss prevention and cognitive decline Fifteen longitudinal studies examining the effect of number of teeth on the subsequent decline of cognitive function or the onset of dementia were assessed. Of the nine reports that focused on the onset of dementia, one was a case–control study (Gatz et al. 2006) and the other eight were cohort studies (Stein et al. 2007; Arrivé et al. 2012; Paganini-Hill et al. 2012; Yamamoto et al. 2012a; Batty et al. 2013; Okamoto et al. 2015; Stewart et al. 2015; Takeuchi et al. 2017). Five of these reports showed that tooth loss was a risk factor for subsequent dementia, two of the remaining three reports (Okamoto et al. 2015; Stewart et al. 2015) did not show a significant relationship, and one report (Arrivé et al. 2012) was contraindicative, indicating that a higher number of lost teeth was associated with a lower risk of onset of dementia. Concerning cognitive decline, six papers have been published (Shimazaki et al. 2001; Kaye et al. 2010; Stein et al. 2010; Naorungroj et al. 2015; Tsakos et al. 2015; Li et al. 2017); four of them (Kaye et al. 2010; Stein et al. 2010; Tsakos et al. 2015; Li et al. 2017) showed significant relationships, but the remaining two (Shimazaki et al. 2001; Naorungroj et al. 2015) did not.

Four studies (Chen et al. 2010; Luo et al. 2015; Bachkati et al. 2017; Takeuchi et al. 2017) have examined the link between cognitive decline or the onset of dementia and number of teeth. In a case–control study that examined the onset of dementia, both the number of lost teeth and the rate of tooth loss were higher in dementia patients, but there was no significant difference (Chen et al. 2010). On the other hand, in a cross-sectional survey of 3063 elderly people in China, the loss of 16 or more teeth was significantly associated with severe cognitive impairment (Luo et al. 2015). In addition, a cohort study of 1566 elderly people in Hisayama-cho, Fukuoka Prefecture in Japan found that those with 19 or fewer remaining teeth were 1.62 times more likely to develop dementia than those with 20 or more remaining teeth (Takeuchi et al. 2017). One cohort study on cognitive decline found that those who had high cognitive function at the age of 50 or 60 tended to have a high number of teeth at the age of 70 (Bachkati et al. 2017). Although no causal relationship can be identified from this study, it is valuable in that it touches on a variable that is missing from most studies that have investigated this relationship: the duration between tooth loss and loss of cognitive function.

If only reports published in 2015 or later are considered, six out of eight of them showed a significant association between cognitive decline and tooth loss (Luo et al. 2015; Okamoto et al. 2015; Stewart et al. 2015; Tsakos et al. 2015; Li et al. 2017; Takeuchi et al. 2017). A 2016 review, for example, found that tooth loss increases the risk of dementia and cognitive decline (Cerutti-Kopplin et al. 2016), and a 2017 paper also reported that tooth loss increases the risk of dementia and Alzheimer's disease (Takeuchi et al. 2017).

A 2017 report showed that poor oral hygiene may lead to a decrease in cognitive function (Gil-Montoya et al. 2017), and a 2018 report found that patients with dementia have significantly lower maximum aperture (i.e. lip movement function is reduced) than MCI patients (Delwel et al. 2018). These symptoms are accompanied by oral hypofunction, such as a mild decline in occlusal force and chewing ability due to loss of teeth. These findings indicate that preventing oral hypofunction from progressing to oral dysfunction, such as swallowing disorders and chewing dysfunction, may exert a preventive effect on cognitive function decline.

The results of recent studies indicate that preventing tooth loss prevents cognitive decline and the onset of dementia. The evidence reviewed here consists only of observational research, which is considered weaker than interventional research. However, there are serious ethical limitations on conducting interventional research on tooth loss (it would involve extracting teeth), so the best way to strengthen the evidence of this relationship is to accumulate and analyse evidence from a wide variety of countries and regions with differing socioeconomic status, healthcare systems, etc.

In nearly every study on the topic since 2015, a significant association has been found between oral health and the onset of dementia. A 2017 review established a significant link between severe periodontal disease and Alzheimer's disease.

3.4.5   Oral health and health promoting factors

Evidence is accumulating that oral health is connected to a number of important health promoting factors, such as diet, nutrition, physical fitness, ADLs, QOL, stress and sleep. The fact that an individual's oral health condition affects food selection and nutrient intake has long been established (Chauncey et al. 1984; Sheiham et al. 2001). Yoshihara et al. (2005) reported that, in a 3-day food survey with 57 people aged 74 years, when the group with 19 or fewer remaining teeth was compared with the group with 20 or more remaining teeth, participants with more teeth were found to have a significantly greater intake of total protein, animal protein, minerals such as vitamin D, B1 and B6, and vegetables. Similarly, Wakai et al. (2010) conducted a 5-year cohort study of 20 366 dentists, finding that tooth loss led to a decrease in vegetable intake and an increase in carbohydrate intake. Moreover, the National Health and Nutrition Survey of the MHLW of Japan (2013) found lower intake of minerals and proteins in people who cannot chew well compared with those with no masticatory problems.

A review of the evidence regarding the relationship between dental/oral health and nutrition reveals that tooth loss is associated with a decrease in food consumption, mainly that of vegetables and fruits, and nutrient intake, mainly vitamins with anti-oxidation effects (Yoshihara et al. 2005; Wakai et al. 2010). Tooth loss is also associated with obesity and weight loss (Marcenes et al. 2003). This association is affected by factors such as age, sex and race. Among the elderly, in particular, associations between tooth loss and a decrease in total energy intake and malnutrition have been observed (Miyazaki et al. 2015b).

Edentulous individuals with full dentures have inferior nutrition intake compared with non-edentulous individuals, but such an association is not observed among those with adequate denture fit who receive regular maintenance. Self-rated oral pain is associated with malnutrition. However, no improvement effects in terms of nutrition intake have been observed as a result of dental prosthesis treatment alone (Suzuki et al. 2018).

Improvements in healthy dietary intake and nutritional status, which require behaviour modification, are difficult to achieve without nutritional guidance. However, based on these findings, it is likely that regular dental maintenance that results in tooth loss prevention, as well as maintenance of denture fit, can decrease the risk of NCDs, prevent malnutrition among the elderly and prevent the decline of ADL, ultimately leading to the extension of HLE.

There is, however, a methodological challenge that must be overcome in future research – namely, that it is difficult to assess causality because observational studies regarding the association between dental/oral health and nutrition have usually relied on a cross-sectional design. Therefore, studies with a higher level of reliability (e.g. cohort studies) need to be conducted in order to accumulate a stronger body of evidence that would clarify the nature of this association.

There is also a great need for research that assesses the effects of improved nutrition through collaboration between dental professionals and other professionals, such as nutritionists, in the context of an intervention study.

Although tooth loss prevention has been shown to be positively associated with diet and nutrition, an RCT study of patients with full dentures reported that prosthetic treatment alone is insufficient. This study provided evidence that prosthetic treatment needs to be accompanied by dietary guidance regarding nutrition and food selection in order to improve dietary behaviour (Chauncey et al. 1984).

Further investigation is required in order to clarify the relationship (and causality) between nutrient intake, which is affected by an individual's oral health status, and subsequent general health.

With regard to exercise, the association of dental/oral health with physical fitness and ADLs has been investigated. The existing research shows that balance, lower limb muscle strength and upper limb muscle strength are associated with occlusal support and chewing ability, and that deterioration of occlusal status causes deterioration of balance and lower limb muscle strength over time (Miyazaki et al. 2015a).

Concerning the association between oral health and rest, communication and QOL, the research indicates that oral health and health-related QOL are significantly correlated, and that the maintenance and promotion of oral health contribute to improved QOL (Naito 2015).

Furthermore, stress and sleep, which are associated with communication and rest, are also associated with oral status. Poor oral health is associated with tooth pain as well as bruxism, which have adverse effects on sleep and stress. Although few reports exist on these factors, rest and communication are thought to be related to survival, ADLs, social participation and QOL, thereby indirectly affecting healthy longevity. An association between stress and amount of sleep and mortality risk has been reported, so research on how oral health is related to these factors would have great public health significance. Therefore, further accumulation of evidence in this area is needed.

However, the interpretation of these results requires that consideration be given to the specific dental treatment interventions employed, as well as the existence of sampling bias. Moreover, the relationship between oral health status and ADLs is believed to be indirect, via a cause-and-effect chain in which nutritional state and physical strength serve as mediating factors. In other words, oral health status affects nutrition, which in turn affects muscle strength, which of course affects mobility and ADLs, including leaving the home for excursions, social activities and the like.

3.4.6   Social determinants of health

Social determinants of health are the 'causes of the causes', requiring us to go upstream to find the underlying factors that inevitably affect the health and behaviour of people. There is a great deal of evidence, including systematic reviews and meta-analyses both in Japan and globally, that higher income and education level (both at the individual and population level) are associated with better oral health conditions and behaviours, confirming the existence of health inequalities (Aida et al. 2015). These social determinants, therefore, interact in complex ways with oral health at all levels (WHO 2010) (Figure 3.4).

Studies conducted in Japan, where dental treatment is covered under the universal health insurance system, reveal similar health inequalities. Health inequalities arise due to variation not only in disease treatment, but also in disease incidence. Accordingly, inequalities are known to exist even if dental examinations are provided free of charge. In addition to ensuring equal access to care, therefore, dental professionals must adopt a people-centred approach, providing explanations and treatment plans that take into account the environment, culture and health literacy of each patient.

In order to improve the health of society as a whole, including those who are uninterested in or unwilling to contribute to the improvement of their own health, it is essential to develop an approach that takes into account the health-related social determinants that exert great, but often indirect, influence on people's health. Clarifying these social determinants of health is an important first step, but we must at the same time begin to put those findings into action more quickly via policies and public health initiatives, evaluate the effectiveness thereof, and thereby move closer to the realization of a society that promotes, improves and maintains the health of everyone in it.

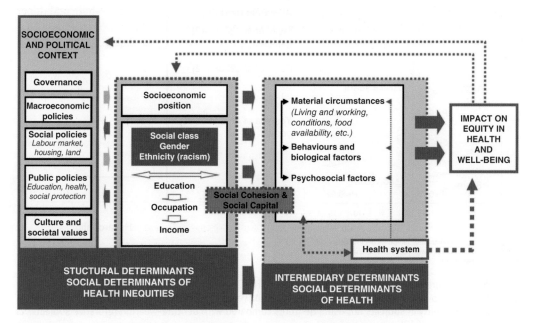

Figure 3.4   Conceptual framework of social determinants of health (WHO 2010).

3.4.7 Effects of dental care and dental management on general health

Cohort studies are beginning to show the effects of dental care for functional recovery and improved oral hygiene on general health.

3.4.7.1 Dental prosthesis and longevity

In a 10-year cohort study in Italy by Appollonio et al. (1997), which consisted of 1137 community residents between the ages of 70 and 75, mortality relative to participants with a sufficient number of natural teeth was 1.3 times higher (HR = 1.34, 95% CI: 1.06–1.70) in those who used dentures and 1.5 times higher (HR = 1.51, 95% CI: 1.11-2.05) in those who had lost teeth but did not use dentures. Another study (Fukai et al. 2008) analysed vital prognosis according to the presence or absence of dental prosthesis while adjusting for number of teeth. This was a 15-year cohort study of 5688 Japanese community residents between the ages 40 and 89, and it provided follow-up results for participants with fewer than 10 functional teeth according to the presence or absence of dental prosthesis. Mortality in women with dentures (HR = 0.72, 95% CI: 0.58–0.91, $P = 0.005$) (Fukai et al. 2008) was 30% lower than in women with no dentures, revealing a clear effect (Figure 3.5).

In addition, some reports propose a relationship between denture use and heart disease, which is a leading cause of death in this population (Polzer et al. 2012; Dai et al. 2022; Liang et al. 2023).

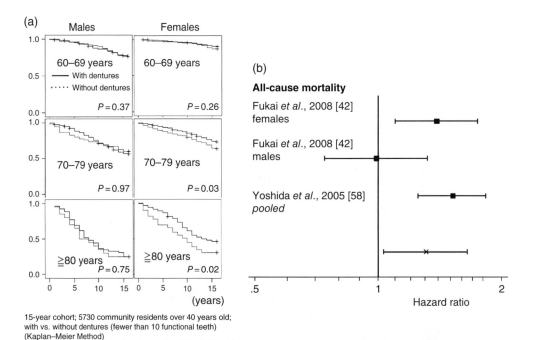

15-year cohort; 5730 community residents over 40 years old;
with vs. without dentures (fewer than 10 functional teeth)
(Kaplan–Meier Method)

Figure 3.5 Denture use and mortality. (a) 15-year cohort, 5730 community residents over 40 years old; females, all age groups; HR = 0.72 (95% CI 0.57–0.91), Cox regression analysis. *Source:* Fukai et al. (2008). (b) All-cause mortality in subjects not using dentures compared with denture-wearing reference subjects. *Source:* Polzer et al. (2012).

3.4.7.2 Dental maintenance and general health

Regarding the effect of dental care on the maintenance of general health and longevity, a significant decrease in tooth loss due to prevention of oral disease and dental management has been established, and there is also sufficient evidence to claim that a decrease in tooth loss prevents the deterioration of general health. In other words, an indirect causal relationship between dental care and general health is supported by sufficient evidence. However, further accumulation of evidence is needed to establish a reliable relationship between improvement in mastication and occlusion and general health maintenance. In addition, further clarification is required regarding the common risk factors of medical, dental and other healthcare fields (e.g. nutrition, personal hygiene, inflammation, smoking).

This chapter has already presented evidence supporting the relationship between oral health and healthy longevity from the perspectives of vital prognosis and the causes of death, avoidance or delay of long-term care, and nutrient intake. In addition to these established relationships, there are a number of other potential areas of association between oral health and general health. The existing evidence needs to be analysed and further studies are needed to investigate these relationships.

A well-known 2-year cohort study conducted by Yoneyama et al. (2002), which included elderly residents of long-term care facilities, confirmed that oral care performed on a regular basis reduced the incidence of pneumonia by about 40%.

Oral health maintenance has been shown to reduce the perioperative complications of surgery. This has important implications not only in terms of improved prognosis but also from the perspective of reducing the economic burden of healthcare services on governments and individuals. Some postoperative complications occur in the oral environment (hygiene status, dental disease, etc.). Therefore, oral management during the perioperative period helps to reduce the risk of infectious complications such as pneumonia, and it contributes to postoperative recovery by supporting the reinitiation of oral intake after surgery. To date, studies have reported evidence regarding risk reduction for the following specific postoperative complications: (1) postoperative pneumonia, (2) complications during endotracheal intubation (tooth fracture and loss, etc.), (3) infection during cardiovascular surgery, (4) infection during organ transplant surgery, and (5) postoperative complications associated with oropharyngeal and oesophageal surgery (respiratory complications, wound infection) (Ueno et al. 2015).

With regard to the effect of dental care on improvement of oral function, there is evidence for the recovery of mastication due to dental prosthesis treatment after tooth loss, significant contribution of improved chewing ability to systemic health, and possible improvements in general health, particularly among the elderly, resulting from the provision of professional care in patients whose oral function has been reduced to the extent that chewing capacity is hindered (Morito et al. 2015).

Many reports have provided evidence that proper continuation of maintenance aimed at preventing the worsening of dental diseases such as dental caries and periodontal disease can help to prevent tooth loss. In these studies, the necessary dental treatment is performed before initiating maintenance, and even during the maintenance period it is necessary to carry out early disease detection and treatment procedures. Long-term preservation of teeth can be achieved through proper dental treatment and continued maintenance. Some reports have indicated that putting a complete veneer crown on teeth that have been subjected to root canal treatment decreases the rate of tooth loss. However, taken together, the results described here show that dental treatment alone does not ensure a sufficient prevention of tooth loss unless maintenance is continued as well (Izumi et al. 2015). In relation to dental disease prevention, topical fluoride applications such as fluoride-containing dentifrices and fluoride mouth rinsing have been shown to be effective in preventing dental caries in primary teeth as well as permanent teeth in young people.

The degree of effectiveness of health guidance and dental health education, particularly regarding participant behaviour modification and oral status improvement, was examined in a review (Yamamoto and Tsuneishi 2015). In addition, paying particular attention to the relationships among risk factors that are common to dental diseases and systemic chronic diseases, Yamamoto and Tsuneishi (2015) conducted a literature search to examine the possibility of dental health education contributing to the common risk factor approach.

However, many of these studies have verified only the short-term effects (i.e. 6 months or less) of dental health education, so the long-term effects are still unclear. Dental healthcare professionals should keep in mind that dental health education is probably effective only for a short-term period of up to 6 months, and they should conduct dental health guidance accordingly. Based on the fact that dental caries and periodontal disease have the characteristics of lifestyle-related diseases and that health education has short-term effects, it is important to encourage patients to visit a dentist regularly, at least every 6 months, and to provide them with dental health guidance during each visit. In order to efficiently carry out dental health education in the field of clinical and public health, there is a need to consider the cost-effectiveness of various types of dental health education. Among the risk factors that are common to dental and systemic health (nutrition, personal hygiene, smoking, drinking, stress and injury), smoking is one where dental health instruction is clearly effective.

3.4.7.3 Dental care and general health promotion

My study of Japanese dental patients – The 8020 Promotion Foundation Study on the health promotion effects of dental care – was conducted to investigate the effect of dental care on maintaining and promoting general health in Japan, which has a national health insurance system and has become a super-ageing society (Fukai et al. 2016, 2017, 2018, 2019, 2021). The study was conducted from 2014 to 2019 with the cooperation of dental patients and dental clinics nationwide.

This project was the first large-scale, nationwide follow-up survey of dental patients in Japan, and probably in the world. There have been few studies to date that have investigated the effect of dental care on general health in the context of a public health insurance system. This study was also viewed as a way to assess the return on investment with regard to the national subsidies that support this system.

This project was a 5-year follow-up study, from 2014 to 2019, in which dental examinations (to determine professionally assessed dental status) were conducted and questionnaires (to determine subjective dental and general health status, self-reported medical history, health behaviour and socioeconomic background) were administered to 12 496 dental patients who visited 1237 dental clinics nationwide during the baseline year, 2014. At baseline, the characteristics of the dental clinics where the examinations were carried out were examined and documented, and a questionnaire was administered to community residents for comparison.

The results of the study are briefly summarized here:

1) Regular dental visitation and tooth loss (Saito et al. 2019)
   - An initial statistical analysis was conducted at the 2-year point of this 5-year follow-up study. Number of teeth lost was set as the dependent variable, and a variety of person-level factors and tooth-level factors were analysed as independent variables via multi-level analysis (generalized estimating equation).

- The number of participants who lost one or more teeth during the first 2-year period was 614 (22.4%). Of the 66 293 teeth present at baseline, 968 (1.5%) were lost. A multi-level analysis using total number of teeth lost as the dependent variable found that smoking habit at baseline and reason for dental visit were significantly associated with tooth loss.
- In other words, the risk of tooth loss in smokers was 1.42 times higher than in non-smokers, and the risk of tooth loss for those who had regular checkups was 39% lower (OR = 0.61) than for those who visited to have a specific dental problem treated.
- Self-reported economic status (income) was also significantly associated with tooth loss, as were a number of indicators of dental status: baseline number of teeth, tooth type, tooth condition and status of periodontal tissue.

2) Oral health instruction, number of dental hygienists, and tooth loss (Saito et al. 2020)
- At the 3-year point of the 5-year follow-up study, a multi-level analysis (generalized estimating equation) was carried out using presence or absence of tooth loss as the dependent variable and clinic-level factors and individual-level (patient-level) factors as independent variables.
- The percentage of participants who lost one or more teeth during the 3-year period was 691 (27.8%). The multi-level analysis showed that, of the clinic-level factors, the duration of oral health instruction and the number of dental hygienists at the dental clinic were significantly associated with tooth loss. Tooth loss risk at dental clinics that provided health guidance of 20 minutes or more was 31% lower than at dental clinics that did not provide oral health instruction, and tooth loss risk at dental clinics with four or more dental hygienists was 33% lower than at dental clinics without dental hygienists.
- Patient-level (individual-level) factors significantly associated with tooth loss were age, baseline number of teeth, average periodontal pocket depth, smoking habit, awareness of bleeding during brushing, and reason for dental visit.

3) Regular dental examinations and tooth loss (Fukai et al. 2021)
- At the 5-year point, the tooth loss of the group receiving only regular dental examinations was compared with the other groups. Of the patients who had been receiving regular checkups for 5 years, 81.0% had no tooth loss, compared with 54.9% for other patients. This indicates that regular dental examination helps to maintain oral health and prevent tooth loss.

A more detailed summary of this study, including the recommendations, is presented in the following sections.

3.4.7.3.1 Dental visitation in Japan (Fukai et al. 2016, 2017) The baseline questionnaire revealed that 76.4% of dental patients (and 63.6% of community residents) had visited a dental clinic within the past year. When dental patients were asked about the reason for their visit to a dental clinic, 57.0% answered that it was for treatment, 30.8% answered that it was for a regular checkup, 12.3% answered that it was for both treatment and a regular checkup. The total percentage of patients visiting for a regular checkup, therefore, was 43.1%.

On the other hand, when community residents were asked about the reason for their last visit to a dental clinic, 35.5% replied that it was for a routine checkup, 7.6 percentage points lower than when dental patients were asked. More than 60% of community residents nationwide had visited a dentist in the past year, and more than one in three indicated that they visited a dentist regularly.

When asked whether they have a regular dental clinic (family dentist), 74.0% of community residents responded in the affirmative. This figure was 55.1% for 20- to 24-year-olds and 88.9% for 75- to 79-year-olds.

These results provide a heretofore unavailable picture of the current state of dental visitation behaviour and dental health maintenance behaviour in Japan.

3.4.7.3.2 Number of teeth and systemic health (baseline data analysis) (Fukai et al. 2016) The association between number of teeth and whole-body health was analysed via cross-sectional analysis of the baseline data.

This analysis found that a higher the number of present teeth was significantly associated with lower prevalence of NCDs, including diabetes mellitus, stroke, heart disease, cancer, hypertension and dyslipidaemia (trend test, $P < 0.05$; χ^2 test, $P < 0.05$).

These results indicated a clear relationship between number of teeth and general physical health.

3.4.7.3.3 Number of teeth and systemic health (follow-up analysis) (Fukai et al. 2018, 2019, 2021) The association between the number of present teeth at baseline and the incidence rate of NCDs during the 5-year period (as well as subjective health deterioration) was analysed (Figure 3.6).

This analysis found that 2.1% of those with 20 or more teeth developed diabetes mellitus, compared with 3.6% of those with 19 teeth or less ($P = 0.009$). Similarly, the incidence rates for those with more versus fewer teeth were 2.3% versus 4.7% ($P < 0.001$) for cancer, 8.2% versus 14.8% ($P < 0.001$) for hypertension, 0.4% and 0.9% ($P = 0.037$) for cerebrovascular accidents, 2.4% versus 4.3% ($P = 0.001$) for heart disease, 6.1% versus 8.6% ($P = 0.009$) for hyperlipidaemia, and 8.2% versus 15.6% ($P < 0.001$) for subjective health conditions (poor).

These results indicated that a higher number of present teeth helps to maintain general physical health due to a suppressive effect on the incidence of NCDs and the deterioration of subjective health conditions.

3.4.7.3.4 Periodontal disease and systemic health (Furuta et al. 2019; Nguyen et al. 2022) A fixed-effect analysis of the association between gingival haemorrhage (as an indicator of periodontal tissue health) and subjective general physical health was conducted, finding that subjective

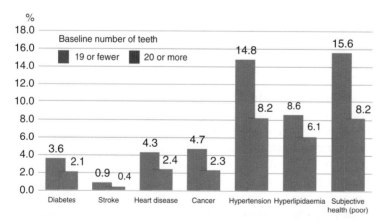

Figure 3.6 Number of teeth and incidence of NCDs and subjective health: 5-year cohort. Baseline participants: 12 278 dental patients at 1215 dental clinics. Analysing the relationship between number of teeth at baseline and general health status 5 years later, the results indicated that those who had 20 or more teeth had a lower incidence of NCDs such as diabetes, cerebrovascular disease, heart disease, cancer, hypertension, and hyperlipidaemia compared with those who had fewer than 20 teeth ($P < 0.01$).
Source: Fukai et al. 2021 / Springer Nature / CCBY 4.0 / Public domain.

physical health status deteriorated as the number of teeth with gingival haemorrhage increased ($B = 0.006$, $P = 0.002$).

In addition, a Poisson regression analysis of patients undergoing regular dental examinations who had past experience of periodontal disease, where having five or more PPD $\geq$ 5 mm teeth was the dependent variable and disease prevalence and obesity were the independent variables, found that diabetes mellitus and hypertension were associated with deep periodontal pockets. This means it is important to pay attention to diabetes mellitus and high blood pressure when providing preventive management of periodontal disease.

3.4.7.3.5 *Factors associated with tooth loss (Fukai et al. 2021)*   The results of a multi-level analysis of the factors related to tooth retention (tooth loss prevention) found that smoking habit at baseline and reason for dental examination were significantly associated with tooth loss.

Specifically, the risk of tooth loss was significantly higher in smokers than in non-smokers (OR = 1.42) and significantly lower in those who visited clinics for regular check-ups than in those who visited for treatment (OR = 0.61). In addition, subjective economic status and number of present teeth were significantly associated with tooth loss. Other factors significantly associated with tooth loss were tooth type, tooth status and periodontal status.

This analysis also revealed a number of dental clinic-related factors that contribute to tooth loss. The duration of oral health guidance provided and the number of dental hygienists at each clinic were significantly associated with tooth loss. Specifically, the risk of tooth loss was significantly lower (OR = 0.69) in dental clinics that provided 20 minutes or more of oral health guidance than at those that did not set aside time for oral health guidance. Tooth loss risk was also significantly lower (OR = 0.67) at dental clinics with four or more dental hygienists than at dental clinics with no dental hygienists.

Other patient characteristics were also significantly associated with tooth loss: age, average periodontal pocket depth, awareness of bleeding during brushing, and reason for dental visit.

3.4.7.3.6 *Oral health maintenance and systemic health (Fukai et al. 2021)*   In order to determine the relationship between regular dental check-ups and systemic health, the incidence rate of NCDs was employed as an indicator of systemic health. This analysis found that the rate of onset of heart disease was significantly lower in patients who had been receiving regular dental examinations continuously for 5 years (1.1%) than in other participants (2.9%) ($P < 0.05$). For hypertension and cancer as well, those who had regular dental examinations for 5 years had a lower onset rate than other patients ($P = 0.057$).

These results indicated that long-term oral health maintenance, including regular dental check-ups, plays an important role in preventing deterioration of systemic health.

3.4.7.3.7 *Effectiveness of regular dental check-ups for tooth loss prevention (Fukai et al. 2021)*   In order to investigate the relationship between regular dental check-ups and tooth loss, the 5-year tooth loss status of participants who were undergoing regular dental examinations was compared with the other participants.

The results of this analysis revealed that 81.0% of the patients who had been receiving regular check-ups for 5 years had no tooth loss, compared with just 54.9% of other participants. This provides evidence that regular dental examinations contribute to prevention of tooth loss and thereby to oral health maintenance.

3.4.7.3.8 *Factors related to regular dental visitation (Fukai et al. 2021; Inoue et al. 2021)*   We also analysed the factors related to dental examination patterns, in both the baseline and follow-up studies. These analyses found that dental clinics employing a higher number of dental hygienists had a higher rate of patients undergoing regular examinations. They also identified two factors that were more common among those who had shifted to a regular dental examination routine: female gender and self-reported economic status at the moderate level or higher.

The relationship between the number of dental hygienists employed at dental clinics and regular dental check-ups by patients was analysed using multiple logistic regression analysis of the baseline data while adjusting for differences among prefectures. The results revealed that even after adjusting for gender, age and economic situation, patients were more likely to undergo regular check-ups at clinics that employed larger numbers of dental hygienists. These results suggest that employing more dental hygienists leads to an increase in regular dental examinations.

Using the 5-year follow-up data, a multi-level logistic regression analysis was performed to identify contributing factors in dental patients who changed their dental visitation pattern from 'for treatment only' to 'for regular dental checkups'. The factors significantly related to transitioning to regular dental visitation were as follows.

Women were 1.30 times more likely than men to shift to regular visitation, and those with high and middle subjective economic status were more likely (1.18 and 1.08 times more likely, respectively) to make that transition than those reporting low economic status. Those with no subjective symptoms were 1.50 times more likely than those with subjective symptoms, and those having completed university education or higher and those having completed secondary education were more likely (1.27 and 1.11 times more likely, respectively) than those who had not completed secondary education. Unemployed people were 1.11 times more likely to shift to regular visitation than employed people. Compared with clinics with no dental hygienists, patients were 2.26 times more likely to shift to regular check-ups at clinics employing more than two dental hygienists, 1.82 times more likely at clinics with 1–1.9 hygienists, and 1.47 times more likely at clinics with 0–0.9 hygienists.

This analysis also clarified that the lower the economic status, the less likely a patient would begin visiting for regular check-ups.

3.4.7.3.9 *Comparison of oral health between community residents and dental patients (Fukai et al. 2021)*
Comparing the results of the survey of general residents with the results of the survey of dental patients, we found that although dental patients tend to receive dental examinations more frequently than the general population, even among the general population more than half of those aged 20–39 and about 70% of those aged 60–79 had visited a dental clinic within the past year.

Regarding self-assessed general health conditions, the data established that the general population felt that some of their health conditions were better compared with dental patients, but there were no significant differences between the two populations in any of the age groups.

In order to compare the general health of dental patients with that of the general population, the prevalence of specific diseases in the two groups was compared by gender. This analysis found no significant difference in the prevalence of diabetes, heart disease, hypertension and dyslipidaemia in men. In women, on the other hand, the prevalence of hypertension was higher among general residents than dental patients for the 20-39 year-old group, but significantly higher in dental patients than in the general population for the age groups 40–59 and 60–29 years.

3.4.7.3.10 *Recommendations*   Based on the results described in the preceding sections, we issued the following recommendations:

1) More than one in three people visit a dentist's office for regular dental check-ups (oral healthcare), and the proportion is increasing among the elderly. In addition, a close look at the content of dental care and health guidance provided at dental clinics reveals that the dental care

provided in Japan is shifting to preventive dental care that responds to the needs of a super-ageing society. In order to further advance this trend, it is necessary to adopt an evidence-based approach to identify and reduce the factors that inhibit dental clinics from transitioning more fully to preventive care.

2) This study provided multiple types evidence for the health promotion effect of dental care. It showed that retention of a greater number of teeth, maintenance of good periodontal status and regular dental check-ups all contribute to preventing the onset of NCDs such as cancer, diabetes and heart disease, as well as the deterioration of the subjective health condition. In other words, it was confirmed that dental care can contribute to the prevention of serious systemic illnesses and diseases, thereby extending HLE. The effect of regular dental check-ups on tooth loss prevention was also clarified. This evidence provides strong justification for further and more detailed investigations into how dental care promotes general public health and stability of the social security system, as well as its medical economic effect.

3) The results of this study provided clear evidence that social and economic factors such as the dental care provision system (including the availability of health guidance and the employment of dental hygienists) and individual socioeconomic status are prominent among the factors contributing to tooth retention, dental disease prevention and regular dental visitation. This indicates a need to reform the national health insurance system to respond to the disparity in dental and oral health access and behaviour.

4) In order to respond to these socioeconomic health disparities, a 'dental public health' approach is required. This would entail the continued and improved prevention of dental diseases and tooth loss in collaboration with local governments via dental care, maintenance and improvement of oral function, but it would also mean a shift towards incorporating general health maintenance and health improvement guidance in dental care settings.

5) To that end, it is necessary to enhance health guidance in dental institutions, and in order to encourage that, there is a need for evidence-based positioning of systemic diseases as risk factors for dental diseases, promotion of medical and dental cooperation in both directions, and reformation of the medical insurance system such that socioeconomic obstacles to dental care access are reduced.

6) Providing high-quality and efficient dental care is essential for improving quality of life and maintaining and promoting health, and it would also contribute to the strengthening and stabilization of the social security system. In order to provide this level of care, policy proposals based on evidence such as real-world data ('big data') and large-scale follow-up studies are required.

7) In order to accumulate such evidence more efficiently, one of the most effective steps would be to establish, ideally on a global scale, a database for monitoring and surveillance of dental care provision and a centralized agency responsible for the prevention and control of dental diseases (tentative name: Dental Centre for Disease Prevention and Control, or DCDC).

8) Due to the clear and direct effect of dental care on general health promotion, governments should invest resources into further developing the public health potential of dental professionals and clinics. A dental public health system could be developed by establishing a new 'dental public health' training and certification programme. The evidence presented herein clearly shows that moving in this direction would have a great effect on healthy longevity.

9) The database containing the baseline data of 12 000 people obtained during this research project, as well as the 5-year follow-up data, represents a valuable resource for obtaining evidence that can be used to justify and implement health promotion activities.

3.5 Conclusion

Based on the evidence and analyses presented in this chapter, the following actions should be prioritized in order to create and sustain a society in which all people can achieve dental and oral health and healthy longevity:

1) A strong body of evidence shows that the prevention of tooth loss contributes to healthy longevity. Through collaborative interprofessional efforts involving medical, dental and community health professionals and institutions, greater efforts should be made to prevent dental diseases (e.g. dental caries and periodontal disease) and the tooth loss that results therefrom.
2) Efforts should be made, from the standpoint of dental health care provision, to accumulate evidence regarding the effects of maintaining and recovering masticatory function and occlusal support, as well as the effect of prevention and control of dental diseases on systemic health.
3) High-quality research should be conducted to accumulate evidence that further clarifies the causal relationship linking dental and oral health to healthy longevity.
4) Research estimating the medical economic effects of dental and oral health policy implementation should be promoted.
5) Evidence-based health policies that reflect the association between dental and oral health and the extension of HLE should be implemented, and studies verifying the effectiveness of these policies should be prioritized.

The realization of the 'society of longevity', which we currently enjoy, represents the achievement of a goal that has been common to societies throughout history and it is the result of centuries of scientific advancement. On the other hand, the decline of vital functions and physical and mental health that is inherent to the ageing process is something we cannot avoid biologically. And the dark side of the ageing coin is that health inequity and injustice persist, not only globally but also within each country, region and city. To address the negative effects of our ageing societies, we need to develop a social structure and healthcare system that reduce both generational and geographical health inequities, thereby allowing both elderly and low-income individuals to lead their lives with purpose and dignity while extending HLE for each and every individual.

Since the implementation of a universal health insurance system in 1961, the health of the people of Japan has improved considerably and the country has achieved a level of longevity greater than anywhere else in the world. As the nation standing at the forefront of the global trend towards longevity, Japan has a responsibility to share the story of its experiences and successes with the world, particularly concerning its healthcare policies and campaigns, even while continuing to reform its own healthcare system.

As the evidence and analyses presented in this chapter confirm, basic dental and oral functionality is associated with self-expression and socialization – which are fundamental human rights – through diet and communication. In the long run, dental and oral health is also associated with overall physical and mental health in general, particularly in terms of prevention and control of NCDs and frailty. In fact, an accumulation of evidence suggests that dental care and oral health are essential contributing factors for the promotion of healthy longevity.

References

Abnet, C.C., Qiao, Y.L., Dawsey, S.M. et al. (2005). Tooth loss is associated with increased risk of total death and death from upper gastrointestinal cancer, heart disease, and stroke in a Chinese population-based cohort. *Int J Epidemiol*, 34, 467–474.

Aida, J., Kondo, K., Yamamoto, T. et al. (2011). Oral health and cancer, cardiovascular, and respiratory mortality of Japanese. *J Dent Res*, 90(9), 1129–1135.

Aida, J., Kondo, K., Hirai, H. et al. (2012). Association between dental status and incident disability in an older Japanese population. *JAGS*, 60, 338–343.

Aida, J., Matsuyama, Y., Koyama, S. et al. (2015). *Oral Health and Social Determinants – Oral Health Inequality and Social Determinants of Oral Health*. The current evidence of dental care and oral health for achieving healthy longevity in an aging society 2015. Japan Dental Association, 216–234.

Aihara, M., Mihara, H., Murayama, T et al. (2010). *GRADE System for Clinical Practice Guideline – Therapeutic Intervention*. Aomori: Topan Publishers.

Albuquerque-Souza, E., & Sahingur, S.E. (2022). Periodontitis, chronic liver diseases, and the emerging oral-gut-liver axis. *Periodontol* 2000, 89(1), 125–141. https://www.ncbi.nlm.nih.gov/pmc/articles/PMC9314012/pdf/PRD-89-125.pdf (accessed 13 May 2024).

Amato, A. (2023,13). Periodontitis and cancer: beyond the boundaries of oral cavity. *Cancers*, 15(6), 1736. https://www.ncbi.nlm.nih.gov/pmc/articles/PMC10046642/pdf/cancers-15-01736.pdf (accessed 13 May 2024).

Ando, A., Tanno, K., Ohsawa, M. et al. (2014). Associations of number of teeth with risks for all-cause mortality and cause-specific mortality in middle-aged and elderly men in the northern part of Japan, The Iwate-KENCO study. *Community Dent Oral Epidemiol*, 42(4), 358–365.

Ansai, T., Takata, Y., Soh, I. et al. (2007). Relationship between chewing ability and 4-year mortality in a cohort of 80-year-old Japanese people. *Oral Dis*, 13(2), 214–219.

Ansai, T., Takata, Y., Soh, I. et al. (2010). Relationship between tooth loss and mortality in 80-year-old Japanese community-dwelling subjects. *BMC Public Health*, 10, 386.

Appollonio, I., Carabellese, C., Frattola, A., & Trabucchi, M. (1997). Dental status, quality of life, and mortality in an older community population, a multivariate approach. *J Am Geriatr Soc*, 45(11), 1315–1323.

Araki, E., Goto, A., Kondo, T. et al. (2020). Japanese Clinical Practice Guideline for Diabetes 2019. *Diabetol Int*, 11(3), 165–223.

Arrivé, E., Letenneur, L., Matharan, F. et al. (2012). Oral health condition of French elderly and risk of dementia: a longitudinal cohort study. *Community Dent Oral Epidemiol*, 40(3), 230–238.

Bachkati, K.H., Mortensen, E.L., Bronnum-Hansen, H., & Holm-Pedersen, P. (2017). Midlife cognitive ability, education, and tooth loss in older Danes. *J Am Geriatr Soc*, 65(1), 194–199.

Barberger-Gateau, P., Letenneur, L. et al. (2002). Fish, meat, and risk of dementia: cohort study. *Br Med J*, 325(7370), 932–933.

Batty, G.D., Li, Q., Huxley, R. et al. & VANCE Collaborative group. (2013). Oral disease in relation to future risk of dementia and cognitive decline: prospective cohort study based on the Action in Diabetes and Vascular Disease: Preterax and Diamicron Modified-Release Controlled Evaluation (ADVANCE) trial. *Eur Psychiatry*, 28(1), 49–52.

Beukers, N.G.F.M., Su, N., Loos, B.G., & van der Heijden, G.J. M.G. (2021). Lower number of teeth is related to higher risks for ACVD and death: systematic review and meta-analyses of survival data. *Front Cardiovasc Med*, 8, 621–626.

Blaschke, K., Hellmich, M., Samel, C. et al. (2022). Association between periodontal treatment and healthcare costs in patients with coronary heart disease: a cohort study based on German claims data. *Dent J*, 10(7), 133. https://www.ncbi.nlm.nih.gov/pmc/articles/PMC9320253/pdf/dentistry-10-00133.pdf (accessed 13 May 2024).

Boaz, A., Davies, H., Fraser, A. & Nutley, S. (2019). *What Works Now? Evidence-Informed Policy and Practice*. Bristol, UK: Bristol University Press.

Botelho, J., Mascarenhas, P., Viana, J. et al. (2022). An umbrella review of the evidence linking oral health and systemic noncommunicable diseases. *Nat Commun*, 13(1), 7614.

Butterfield, D., Castegna, A., Pocernich, C. et al. (2002). Nutritional approaches to combat oxidative stress in Alzheimer's disease. *J Nutr Biochem*, 13(8), 444.

Cabrera, C., Hakeberg, M., Ahlqwist, M. et al. (2005). Can the relation between tooth loss and chronic disease be explained by socio-economic status? A 24-year follow-up from the population study of women in Gothenburg, *Sweden. Eur J Epidemiol*, 20(3), 229–236.

Cardoso, A.F., Ribeiro, L.E., Santos, T. et al.(2023). Oral hygiene in patients with stroke: a best practice implementation project protocol. *Nurs Rep*, 13(1), 148–156.

Cerutti-Kopplin, D., Feine, J et al. (2016). Tooth loss increases the risk of diminished cognitive function: a systematic review and meta-analysis. *JDR Clin & Transl Res*, 1(1), 10–19.

Cestari, J.A., Fabri, G.M., Kalil, J. et al. (2016). Oral infections and cytokine levels in patients with Alzheimer's disease and mild cognitive impairment compared with controls. *J Alzheimers Dis*, 52(4), 1479–1485.

Chauncey, H.H., Muench, M.E., Kapur, K.K., & Wayler, A.H. (1984). The effect of the loss of teeth on diet and nutrition. *Int Dent J*, 34(2), 98–104.

Chen, Z.Y., Chiang, C.H., Huang, C.C. et al. (2012). The association of tooth scaling and decreased cardiovascular disease: a nationwide population-based study. *Am J Med*, 125, 568–575.

Chen, C.K., Wu, Y.T., & Chang, Y.C. (2017). Association between chronic periodontitis and the risk of Alzheimer's disease: a retrospective, population-based, matched-cohort study. *Alzheimers Res Ther*, 9(1), 56.

Chen, H., Nie, S., Zhu, Y., & Lu, M. (2015). Teeth loss, teeth brushing and esophageal carcinoma: a systematic review and meta-analysis. *Sci Rep*, 5, 15203.

Chen, X., Shuman, S.K., Hodges, J.S. et al. (2010). Patterns of tooth loss in older adults with and without dementia: a retrospective study based on a Minnesota cohort. *J Am Geriatr Soc*, 58(12), 2300–2307.

Christensen, K., Doblhammer, G., Rau, R., & Vaupel, J.W. (2009). Ageing populations, the challenges ahead. *Lancet*, 374, 1196–1208.

Dai, J., Li, A., Liu, Y. et al. (2022). Denture wearing status, cardiovascular health profiles, and mortality in edentulous patients: a prospective study with a 27-year follow-up. *J Dent*, 126, 104287.

Delwel, S., Scherder, E.J. A., Perez, R.S.G.M. et al. (2018). Oral function of older people with mild cognitive impairment or dementia. *J Oral Rehabil*, 45(12), 990–997.

Demmer, R.T., Jacobs, D.R. Jr., & Desvarieux, M. (2008). Periodontal disease and incident type 2 diabetes: results from the First National Health and Nutrition Examination Survey and its epidemiologic follow-up study. *Diab Care*, 31(7), 1373–1379.

Demmer, R.T., Desvarieux, M., Holtfreter, B. et al. (2010, May). Periodontal status and A1C change, longitudinal results from the study of health in Pomerania(SHIP). *Diab Care*, 33(5), 1037–1043.

Demmer, R.T., Squillaro, A., Papapanou, P.N. et al. (2012). Periodontal infection, systemic inflammation, and insulin resistance, results from the continuous National Health and Nutrition Examination Survey(NHANES)1999–2004. *Diab Care*, 35(11), 2235–2242.

Dibello, V., Zupo, R., Sardone, R., Bortone, I., Lampignano, L., Giannelli, G., & Panza, F. (2021). Oral frailty and its determinants in older age: a systematic review. *Lancet Healthy Longev*, 2, e507–20.

Dibello, V., Lobbezoo, F., Lozupone, M. et al. (2023). Oral frailty indicators to target major adverse health-related outcomes in older age: a systematic review. *Geroscience*, 45(2), 663–706.

Dietrich, T., Webb, I., Stenhouse, L. et al. (2017). Evidence summary: the relationship between oral and cardiovascular disease. *Br Dent J*, 222(5), 381–385. https://pubmed.ncbi.nlm.nih.gov/28281612/ (accessed 13 May 2024).

Engebretson, S., Kocher, T. (2013). Evidence that periodontal treatment improves diabetes outcomes: a systematic review and meta-analysis. *J Periodontol*, 84(4 Suppl), S153–169.

Evidence-Based Medicine Working Group (1992). Evidence-based medicine. A new approach to teaching the practice of medicine. *J Am Med Assoc*,268(17), 2420–2425.

Fang, W.L., Jiang, M.J., Gu, B.B. et al. (2018). Tooth loss as a risk factor for dementia: systematic review and meta-analysis of 21 observational studies. *BMC Psychiatry*, 18(1), 345.

Fried, L.P., Tangen, C.M., Walston, J. et al. (2001). Cardiovascular Health Study Collaborative Research Group. Frailty in older adults: evidence for a phenotype. *J Gerontol A Biol Sci Med Sci*, 56(3), M146–156.

Fries, J.F. (1980). Aging, natural death, and the compression of morbidity. *N Engl J Med*, 303,130–135.

Fujinami, Y., Hifumi, T., Ono, Y. et al. (2021). Malocclusion of molar teeth is associated with activities of daily living loss and delirium in elderly critically ill older patients. *J Clin Med*, 10(10), 2157.

Fukai, K., Takiguchi, T., Ando, Y. et al. (2007). Functional tooth number and 15-year mortality in a cohort of community-residing older people, *Geriatr Gerontol Int*, 7, 341–347.

Fukai, K., Takiguchi, T., Ando, Y. et al. (2008). Mortalities of community-residing adult residents with and without dentures. *Geriatr Gerontol Int*, 8, 152–159.

Fukai, K., Takiguchi, T., Ando, Y. et al. (2009). Associations between functional tooth number and physical complaints of community residing adults in a 15-year cohort study. *Geriatr Gerontol Int*, 9, 366–371.

Fukai, K., Takiguchi, T., & Sasaki, H. (2010). Dental health and longevity. *Geriatr Gerontol Int*, 10, 275–276.

Fukai, K., Takiguchi, T., Ando, Y. et al. (2011). Critical tooth number without subjective dysphagia. *Geriatr Gerontol Int*, 11, 482–487.

Fukai, K. (2013). Future directions for research on the contributions of dental and oral health to a healthy aging society. *Health Sci Health Care*, 13, 39–42

Fukai, K., Furuta, M., Aida, J. et al. (2016). The oral health and general health of Japanese dental patients: results from the baseline data of the 8020 Promotion Foundation. The study on the health promoting effect of dental care. *J Jap Assoc Dental Sci (JJADS)*, 35, 39–50.

Fukai, K., Furuta, M., Shimazaki, Y. et al. (2017). The oral health and general health of Japanese community residents: The 8020 Promotion Foundation Study on the health promotion effects of dental care. *J Jap Assoc Dental Sci (JJADS)*, 36, 62–73.

Fukai, K., Shimazaki, Y., Furuta, M. et al. T. (2018). Association between oral health and general health of Japanese dental patient: The 8020 Promotion Foundation Study on the health promotion effects of dental care – a 2-year Cohort Study. *J Jap Assoc Dental Sci (JJADS)*, 37, 63–67.

Fukai, K. (2018). Number of functional teeth and 25-year mortality in a cohort of community-residing people. KAKEN.

Fukai, K., Furuta, M., Aida, J. et al. (2019). Association between oral health and general health of Japanese dental patients: The 8020 Promotion Foundation Study on the health promotion effects of dental care – a 3-year cohort study. *J Jap Assoc Dental Sci (JJADS)*, 38, 84–93.

Fukai, K., Furuta, M., Shimazaki, Y. et al. (2021). Association between oral health and general health in Japanese dental patients: The 8020 Promotion Foundation Study on the health promotion effects of dental care: a 5-year cohort study. *J Jap Assoc Dental Sci (JJADS)*, 40, 82–95.

Fukai, K., Dartevelle, S., Jones, J. (2022). Oral health for healthy ageing: a people-centred and function-focused approach. *Int Dent*, 72(4S), S2–S4.

Fukui, T., Yoshida, M., Yamaguchi, N. (2014). *Minds Guideline*. Tokyo: Igakusyoin. https://minds.jcqhc. or.jp/docs/minds/guideline/pdf/handbook2014_0_1.1.pdf (accessed 13 May 2024).

Furuta, M., Fukai, K., Aida, J et al. (2019). Periodontal status and self-reported systemic health of periodontal patients regularly visiting dental clinics in the 8020 Promotion Foundation Study of Japanese Dental Patients. *J Oral Sci*, 61(2), 238–245.

Furuta, M., Komiya-Nonaka, M., Akifusa, S. et al. (2013). Interrelationship of oral health status, swallowing function, nutritional status, and cognitive ability with activities of daily living in Japanese elderly people receiving home care services due to physical disabilities. *Community Dent Oral Epidemiol*, 41(2), 173–181.

Gao, S., Tian, J., Li, Y. et al. (2021). Periodontitis and number of teeth in the risk of coronary heart disease: an updated meta-analysis. *Med Sci Monit*, 27, e930112. https://www.ncbi.nlm.nih.gov/pmc/articles/PMC8394608/pdf/medscimonit-27-e930112.pdf (accessed 13 May 2024).

Gatz, M., Mortimer, J.A., Fratiglioni, L. et al. (2006). Potentially modifiable risk factors for dementia in identical twins. *Alzheimers Dement*, 2(2), 110–117.

Gil-Montoya, J.A., Sánchez-Lara, I., Carnero-Pardo, C. et al. (2017). Oral hygiene in the elderly with different degrees of cognitive impairment and dementia. *J Am Geriatr Soc*, 65(3), 642–647.

Graziani, F., Gennai, S., Solini, A., & Petrini, M. (2018). A systematic review and meta-analysis of epidemiologic observational evidence on the effect of periodontitis on diabetes: An update of the EFP-AAP review. *J Clin Periodontol*, 45(2), 167–187.

Gray, J.A. *Evidence -based Healthcare*. Edinburgh: Churchill Livingstone, 1997.

Guo, Z., Gu, C., Li, S. et al. (2021). Periodontal disease and the risk of prostate cancer: a meta-analysis of cohort studies. *Int Braz J Urol*, 47(6), 1120–1130. https://www.ncbi.nlm.nih.gov/pmc/articles/PMC8486441/pdf/1677–6119-ibju-47–06-1120.pdf (accessed 13 May 2024).

Hanada, N., & Nomura Y. (2015). Association between oral health and main illnesses underlying conditions that necessitate long-term care: articular diseases, periodontal disease and rheumatoid arthritis. *The Current Evidence of Dental Care and Oral Health for Achieving Healthy Longevity in an Aging Society*. Japan Dental Association (Fukai K editor in chief). Japan Dental Association, 162–167.

Hanioka, T., Ojima, M., Tanaka, K. et al. Causal assessment of smoking and tooth loss: a systematic review of observational studies. *BMC Public Health*, 11, 221.

Hashimoto, S. (2014). Study on the analysis and analytical assessment of the current status of healthy life expectancy in Japan and other countries (in Japanese). Tokyo: MHLW. http://toukei.umin.jp/kenkoujyumyou/houkoku/H26_toku.pdf (accessed 8 July 2024).

Hayasaka, K., Tomata, Y., Aida, J. et al. (2013, May). Tooth loss and mortality in elderly Japanese adults: effect of oral care. *J Am Geriatr Soc*, 61(5), 815–820.

Hayflick, L., Moorhead, P.S. (1961). The serial cultivation of human diploid cell strains. *Exp Cell Res*, 25, 585–621.

Hiraki, A., Matsuo, K., Suzuki, T. et al. (2008). Teeth loss and risk of cancer at 14 common sites in Japanese. *Cancer Epidemiol Biomarkers Prev*, 17(5), 1222–1227.

Holm-Pedersen, P., Schultz-Larsen, K., Christiansen, N., & Avlund, K. (2008). Tooth loss and subsequent disability and mortality in old age. *J Am Geriatr Soc*, 56, 429–435.

Holmlund, A., Holm, G., & Lind, L. (2010) Number of teeth as a predictor of cardiovascular mortality in a cohort of 7,674 subjects followed for 12 years. *J Periodontol*, 81(6), 870–876.

Horie, N.C., Serrao, V.T., Simon, S.S. et al. (2016). Cognitive effects of intentional weight loss in elderly obese individuals with mild cognitive impairment. *J Clin Endocrinol Metab*, 101(3), 1104–1112.

Ide, M., Harris, M., Stevens, A. et al. (2016). Periodontitis and cognitive decline in Alzheimer's disease. *PloS One*, 11(3), e0151081.

Ikeda, N., Saito, E., Kondo, N. et al. (2011), What has made the population of Japan healthy? *Lancet*, 378 (9796), 1094–1105.

Inoue, Y., Shimazaki, Y., Oshiro, A. et al. (2021). Multilevel analysis of the association of dental-hygienist-related factors on regular dental check-up behavior. *Int J Environ Res Public Health*, 18(6), 2816.

Ishikawa, S., Konta, T., Susa, S. et al. (2020). Association between presence of 20 or more natural teeth and all-cause, cancer-related, and cardiovascular disease-related mortality: Yamagata (Takahata) prospective observational study. *BMC Oral Health*, 20(1), 353.

Ishimaru, M., Matsui, H., Ono, S. et al. (2018). Preoperative oral care and effect on postoperative complications after major cancer surgery. *Br J Surg*, 105(12), 1688–1696.

Iwai-Saito, K., Shobugawa, Y., Aida, J., Kondo, K. (2021). Frailty is associated with susceptibility and severity of pneumonia in older adults (A JAGES multilevel cross-sectional study). *Sci Rep*, 11(1), 7966.

Iwasaki, M., Hirano, H., Motokawa, K. et al. (2021). Interrelationships among whole-body skeletal muscle mass, masseter muscle mass, oral function, and dentition status in older Japanese adults. *BMC Geriatr*, 21(1), 582.

Iwasaki, M., Yoshihara, A., Kimura, Y. et al. (2016). Longitudinal relationship of severe periodontitis with cognitive decline in older Japanese. *J Periodontal Res*, 51(5), 681–688.

Izumi, Y., Aoyama, N., Matsuura, T., & Mizutani, K. (2015). Preventive effects on tooth loss. *The Current Evidence of Dental Care and Oral Health for Achieving Healthy Longevity in an Aging Society.* Japan Dental Association (Fukai K editor in chief), 252–257.

Janket, S.J., Wightman, A., Baird, A.E. et al. (2005). Does periodontal treatment improve glycemic control in diabetic patients? A meta-analysis of intervention studies. *J Dent Res*, 84, 1154–1159.

Janket, S.J., Baird, A.E., Chuang, S.K., Jones JA. (2003). Meta-analysis of periodontal disease and risk of coronary heart disease and stroke. *Oral Surg Oral Med Oral Pathol Oral Radiol Endod*, 95(5), 559–569.

Japan Dental Association (2016). Dental Medical Awareness Survey. JDA. https://www.jda.or.jp/pdf/DentalMedicalAwarenessSurvey_h28.pdf (accessed 13 May 2024).

Katagiri, S., Nitta, H., Nagasawa, T. et al. (2013). Effect of glycemic control on periodontitis in type 2 diabetic patients with periodontal disease. *J Diabetes Investig*, 4(3), 320–325.

Kaye, E.K., Valencia, A., Baba, N. et al. (2010). Tooth loss and periodontal disease predict poor cognitive function in older men. *J Am Geriatr Soc*, 58(4), 713–718.

Kesharani, P., Kansara, P., Kansara, T. et al. (2022). Is periodontitis a risk factor for lung cancer? A meta-analysis and detailed review of mechanisms of association. *Contemp Clin Dent*, 13(4), 297–306. https://www.ncbi.nlm.nih.gov/pmc/articles/PMC9855255/pdf/CCD-13-297.pdf (accessed 13 May 2024).

Khader, Y.S., Daoud, A.S., El-Qaderi, S.S. et al. (2006). Periodontal status of diabetics compared with nondiabetics, a meta-analysis. *J Diabetes Complications*, 20, 59–68.

Khader, Y.S., Albashaireh, Z.S., Alomari, M.A. (2004). Periodontal diseases and the risk of coronary heart and cerebrovascular diseases: a meta-analysis. *J Periodontol*, 75(8), 1046–1053.

Kikutani, T., Yoneyama, T., Nishiwaki, K. et al. (2010). Effect of oral care on cognitive function in patients with dementia. *Geriatr Gerontol Int*, 10(4), 327–328.

Kimura, H., Kanzaki, N. (2014). Study on cognitive function and mouth care of the elderly at home. *Journal of Japanese Society for Dementia Care*, 13(3), 20.

Kotronia, E., Brown, H., Papacosta, A.O. et al. (2021). Oral health and all-cause, cardiovascular disease, and respiratory mortality in older people in the UK and USA. *Sci Rep*, 11(1), 16452.

Lee, H.J., Choi, E.K., Park, J.B. et al. (2019). Tooth loss predicts myocardial infarction, heart failure, stroke, and death. *J Dent Res*, 98(2), 164–170.

Lee, Y.T., Lee, H.C., Hu, C.J. et al. (2017a). Periodontitis as a modifiable risk factor for dementia: a nationwide population-based cohort study. *J Am Geriatr Soc*, 65(2), 301–305.

Lee, Y.L., Hu, H.Y., Huang, L.Y. et al. (2017b). Periodontal disease associated with higher risk of dementia: population-based cohort study in Taiwan. *J Am Geriatr Soc*, 65(9), 1975–1980.

Leira, Y., Domínguez, C., Seoane, J. et al. (2017). Is periodontal disease associated with Alzheimer's Disease? A systematic review with meta-analysis. *Neuroepidemiology*, 48(1-2), 21–31.

Li, J., Xu, H., Pan, W., & Wu, B. (2017). Association between tooth loss and cognitive decline: a 13-year longitudinal study of Chinese older adults. *PloS One*, 12(2), e0171404.

Liang, X., Chou, O.H.I., & Cheung, B.M.Y. (2023). The association between denture use and cardiovascular diseases. The United States National Health and Nutrition Examination Survey 2009–2018. *Front Cardiovasc Med*, 9, 1000478.

Liljestrand, L.M., Havulinna, A.S., Paju, S. et al. (2015). Missing teeth predict incident cardiovascular events, diabetes, and death. *J Dent Res*, 94(8), 1055–1062.

Lourida, I., Soni, M., Thompson-Coon, J. et al. (2013). Mediterranean diet, cognitive function, and dementia: a systematic review. *Epidemiology*, 24(4), 479–489.

Luo, J., Wu, B., Zhao, Q. et al. (2015). Association between tooth loss and cognitive function among 3063 Chinese older adults: a community-based study. *PloS One*, 10(3), e0120986.

Lynn, J. (2001). Serving patients who may die soon and their families. The role of hospice and other services. *J Am Med Assoc*, 285(7), 925–932.

Machado, V., Aguilera, E.M., Botelho, J. et al. (2020). Association between periodontitis and high blood pressure: results from the Study of Periodontal Health in Almada-Seixal (SoPHiAS). *J Clin Med*. PMID: 32456145

Maekawa, K., Ikeuchi, T., Shinkai, S. et al. (2020). Number of functional teeth more strongly predicts all-cause mortality than number of present teeth in Japanese older adults. *Geriatr Gerontol Int*, 20(6), 607–614.

Marcenes, W., Steele, J.G., Sheiham, A., & Walls, A.W. (2003). The relationship between dental status, food selection, nutrient intake, nutritional status, and body mass index in older people. *Cad Saude Publica*, 19(3), 809–816.

Mascari, R., Vezzeti, A., Orofino, C. et al. (2021). Periodontal disease association with large-artery atherosclerotic stroke. *J Neurol Disord Stroke*, 8(1), 1173.

Matsubara, C., Shirobe, M., Furuya, J. et al. (2021). Effect of oral health intervention on cognitive decline in community-dwelling older adults: a randomized controlled trial. *Arch Gerontol Geriatr*, 92, 104267.

Mattson, M.P., Chan, S.L., & Duan, W. (2002). Modification of brain aging and neurodegenerative disorders by genes, diet, and behavior. *Physiol Rev*, 82(3), 637–672.

Minakuchi, S., Tsuga, K., Ikebe, K. et al. (2018). Oral hypofunction in the older population: position paper of the Japanese Society of Gerodontology in 2016. *Gerodontology*, 35(4), 317–324.

Ministry of Health, Labour and Welfare of Japan (MHLW) (2022). *The 23rd Life Tables in 2020*. Tokyo: MHLW. https://www.mhlw.go.jp/english/database/db-hw/lifetb23nd/dl/data.pdf (accessed 13 May 2024).

Ministry of Health, Labour and Welfare (MHLW) of Japan (2021). *Portal Site of Statistics of Japan*. Tokyo: MHLW.

Ministry Health, Labour and Welfare (MHLW) of Japan (2020). *Long-term Care in 2020*. Tokyo: MHLW.

Ministry of Health, Labour and Welfare (MHLW) of Japan (2019). *Comprehensive Survey of Living Conditions*. Tokyo: MHLW.

Ministry Health Labour and Welfare (MHLW) of Japan (2013). *National Health and Nutrition Survey*. Tokyo: MHLW.

Miyazaki, H., Yamaga, T., & Hanada, N. (2015a). Exercise (including ADL) – oral health, physical fitness and ADL among the elderly. *The Current Evidence of Dental Care and Oral Health for Achieving Healthy Longevity in an Aging Society*. Japan Dental Association (Fukai K editor in chief), 178–188.

Miyazaki, H., Iwasaki, M., Yoshihara, A., Ando, Y. (2015b). Nutrition-dental/oral health and nutrition. *The Current Evidence of Dental Care and Oral Health for Achieving Healthy Longevity in an Aging Society*. Japan Dental Association (Fukai K editor in chief), 190–202.

Morita, I., Nakagaki, H., Kato, K. et al. (2006). Relationship between survival rates and numbers of natural teeth in an elderly Japanese population. *Gerodontology*, 23, 214–218.

Morita, T., Yamazaki, Y., Mita, A. et al. (2010). Cohort study on the association between periodontal disease and the development of metabolic syndrome. *J Periodontol*, 81(4), 512–519.

Morita, I., Inagaki, K., Nakamura, F. et al. (2012). Relationship between periodontal status and levels of glycated hemoglobin. *J Dent Res*, 91(2), 161–166.

Morito, M., & Sato, Y. (2015). Oral function deterioration prevention and recovery. *The Current Evidence of Dental Care and Oral Health for Achieving Healthy Longevity in an Aging Society*. Japan Dental Association (Fukai K editor in chief). Japan Dental Association, 246–250

Morris, M.C., Evans, D.A., Bienias, J.L. et al. (2003). Consumption of fish and n-3 fatty acids and risk of incident Alzheimer disease. *Arch Neurol*, 60(7), 940–946.

Müller, F. (2015). Oral hygiene reduces the mortality from aspiration pneumonia in frail elders. *J Dent Res*, 94(3 Suppl):14S–16S.

Nagatani, M., Tanaka, T., Son, B.K. et al. (2023). Oral frailty as a risk factor for mild cognitive impairment in community-dwelling older adults: Kashiwa study. *Exp Gerontol*, 172, 112075.

Naito, M. (2015). Rest, communication and QOL. *The Current Evidence of Dental Care and Oral Health for Achieving Healthy Longevity in an Aging Society*. Japan Dental Association (Fukai K editor in chief). Japan Dental Association, 204–213.

Naorungroj, S., Schoenbach, V.J., Wruck, L. et al. (2015). Tooth loss, periodontal disease, and cognitive decline in the Atherosclerosis Risk in Communities (ARIC) study. *Community Dent Oral Epidemiol*, 43(1), 47–57.

Naorungroj, S., Slade, G.D., Beck, J.D. et al. (2013). Cognitive decline and oral health in middle-aged adults in the ARIC study. *J Dent Res*, 92(9), 795–801.

Nascimento, G.G., Leite, F.R., Conceição, D.A. et al. (2016). A systematic review and meta-analysis. *Obes Rev*, 17(7):587–98.

National Institute of Population and Social Security Research. (2022). Social Security Expenditure by category, fiscal years 2022 (in Japanese). https://www.ipss.go.jp/ss-cost/j/fsss-R02/fsss_R02.html (accessed 13 May 2024).

Nguyen, V.T.N., Furuta, M., Zaitsu, T. et al. (2022). Periodontal health predicts self-rated general health: A time-lagged cohort study. *Community Dent Oral Epidemiol*, 50(5), 421–429.

Noble, J.M., Scarmeas, N., Celenti, R.S. et al. (2014). Serum IgG antibody levels to periodontal microbiota are associated with incident Alzheimer disease. *PLoS One*, 9(12), e114959.

Nwizu, N., Wactawski-Wende, J., & Genco RJ. (2020). Periodontal disease and cancer: Epidemiologic studies and possible mechanisms. *Periodontol 2000*, 83(1), 213–233. https://www.ncbi.nlm.nih.gov/pmc/articles/PMC7328760/pdf/PRD-83-213.pdf (accessed 13 May 2024).

Okamoto, N., Morikawa, M., Tomioka, K. et al. (2015). Association between tooth loss and the development of mild memory impairment in the elderly: the Fujiwara-kyo Study. *J Alzheimers Dis*, 44(3), 777–786.

Olshansky, S.J., Carnes, B.A., & Cassel, C. (1990). In search of Methuselah, estimating the upper limits to human longevity. *Science*, 250, 634–640.

Osterberg, T., Carlsson, G.E., Sundh, V., & Mellström, D. (2008). Number of teeth – a predictor of mortality in 70-year-old subjects. *Community Dent Oral Epidemiol*, 36(3), 258–268.

Otake, M., Ono, S., Watanabe, Y. et al. (2022). Association between the number of remaining teeth and body mass index in Japanese inpatients with schizophrenia. *Neuropsychiatr Dis Treat*, 18, 2591–2597.

Ozawa, M., Ninomiya, T., Ohara, T. et al. (2013). Dietary patterns and risk of dementia in an elderly Japanese population: the Hisayama Study. *Am J Clin Nutr*, 97(5), 1076–1082.

Ozawa, M., Ohara, T., Ninomiya, T. et al. (2014). Milk and dairy consumption and risk of dementia in an elderly Japanese population: the Hisayama Study. *J Am Geriatr Soc*, 62(7), 1224–1230.

Padilha, D.M., Hilgert, J.B., Hugo, F.N. et al. (2008, July). Number of teeth and mortality risk in the Baltimore Longitudinal Study of Aging. *J Gerontol A Biol Sci Med Sci*, 63(7), 739–744.

Paganini-Hill, A., White, S.C., & Atchison, K.A. (2012). Dentition, dental health habits, and dementia: the Leisure World Cohort Study. *J Am Geriatr Soc*, 60(8), 1556–1563.

Peng, J., Song, J., Han, J. et al. (2019). The relationship between tooth loss and mortality from all causes, cardiovascular diseases, and coronary heart disease in the general population: systematic review and dose-response meta-analysis of prospective cohort studies. *Biosci Rep*, 9(1), BSR20181773.

Polzer, I., Schwahn, C., Völzke, H. et al. (2012). The association of tooth loss with all-cause and circulatory mortality. Is there a benefit of replaced teeth? A systematic review and meta-analysis. *Clin Oral Investig*, 16(2), 333–351. https://pubmed.ncbi.nlm.nih.gov/22086361/ (accessed 13 May 2024).

Rivière, S., Gillette-Guyonnet, S., Voisin, T. et al. (2001). A nutritional education program could prevent weight loss and slow cognitive decline in Alzheimer's disease. *J Nutr Health Aging*, 5(4), 295–299.

Robertson, T.L., Kato, H., Gordon, T. et al. (1977). Epidemiologic studies of coronary heart disease and stroke in Japanese men living in Japan, Hawaii and California. Coronary heart disease risk factors in Japan and Hawaii. *Am J Cardiol*, 39(2), 244–249.

Saito, M., Shimazaki, Y., Fukai, K. et al. (2019). Risk factors for tooth loss in adult Japanese dental patients: 8020 Promotion Foundation Study. *J Investig Clin Dent*, 10(2), e12392.

Saito, M., Shimazaki, Y., Fukai, K. et al. (2020). A multilevel analysis of the importance of oral health instructions for preventing tooth loss: The 8020 Promotion Foundation Study of Japanese Dental Patients. *BMC Oral Health*, 20(1), 328.

Sanz, M., Marco, Del Castillo, A., Jepsen, S. et al. (2020). Periodontitis and cardiovascular diseases: Consensus report. *J Clin Periodontol*, 47(3), 268–288

Sasaki, H. (2008). Single pathogenesis of geriatric syndrome. *Geriatr Gerontol Int*, 8(1), 1–4.

Scarmeas, N., Stern, Y., Tang, M.X. et al. (2006). Mediterranean diet and risk for Alzheimer's disease. *Ann Neurol*, 59(6), 912–921.

Schroeder, S.A. (2007). We can do better-improving the health of the American people. *New Engl J Med*, 357(12), 1221–1228.

Schwahn, C., Polzer, I., Haring, R. et al. (2013). Missing, unreplaced teeth and risk of all-cause and cardiovascular mortality. *Int J Cardiol*, 167(4), 1430–7.

Seko, R., Hashimoto, S., Kawado, M. et al. (2012). Trends in life expectancy with care needs based on long-term care insurance data in Japan. *J Epidemiol*, 22(3), 238–243.

Sen, S., Giamberardino, L.D., Moss, K. et al. (2018). Periodontal disease, regular dental care use, and incident ischemic stroke. *Stroke*, 49(2), 355–362.

Sen, S., & Mascari, R. (2020). Exploring the periodontal disease-ischemic stroke link. *J Periodontol*, 91 Suppl 1, S35–S39.

Sfyroeras, G.S., Roussas, N., Saleptsis, V.G. et al. (2012). Association between periodontal disease and stroke. *J Vasc Surg*, 55(4), 1178–1184.

Shah, R. (2013). The role of nutrition and diet in Alzheimer disease: a systematic review. *J Am Med Dir Assoc*, 14(6), 398–402.

Sheiham, A., & Watt, R.G. (2000). The common risk factor approach: a rational basis for promoting oral health. *Community Dent Oral Epidemiol*, 28(6), 399–406.

Sheiham, A., Steele, J.G., Marcenes, W. et al. (2001). The relationship among dental status, nutrient intake, and nutritional status in older people. *J Dent Res*, 80(2), 408–413.

Shi, J., Leng, W., Zhao, L. et al. (2017). Tooth loss and cancer risk: a dose–response meta analysis of prospective cohort studies. *Oncotarget*, 9(19), 15 090–15 100.

Shimazaki, Y., Soh, I., Saito, T. et al. (2001). Influence of dentition status on physical disability, mental impairment, and mortality in institutionalized elderly people. *J Dent Res*, 80(1), 340–345.

Shirobe, M., Watanabe, Y., Tanaka, T. et al. (2021, July 9). Effect of an oral frailty measures program on community-dwelling elderly people: a cluster-randomized controlled trial. *Gerontology*, 68(4), 377–386.

Simpson, T.C., Weldon, J.C., Worthington, H.V. et al. (2015). Treatment of periodontal disease for glycaemic control in people with diabetes mellitus. *Cochrane Database Syst Rev*, 2015(11),

Singh, B., Parsaik, A.K., Mielke, M.M. et al. (2014). Association of Mediterranean diet with mild cognitive impairment and Alzheimer's disease: a systematic review and meta-analysis. *J Alzheimers Dis*, 39(2), 271–282.

Stein, P. S, Kryscio R.J., Desrosiers, M. et al. (2010). Tooth loss, apolipoprotein E, and decline in delayed word recall. *J Dent Res*, 89(5), 473–477.

Stein, P.S., Desrosiers, M., Donegan, S.J. et al. (2007). Tooth loss, dementia and neuropathology in the Nun study. *J Am Dent Assoc*, 138(10), 1314–1322.

Stewart, R., Stenman, U., Hakeberg, M. et al. (2015). Associations between oral health and risk of dementia in a 37-year follow-up study: the prospective population study of women in Gothenburg. *J Am Geriatr Soc*, 63(1), 100–105.

Suzuki, H., Kanazawa, M., Komagamine, Y. et al. (2018). The effect of new complete denture fabrication and simplified dietary advice on nutrient intake and masticatory function of edentulous elderly: a randomized-controlled trial. *Clin Nutr*, 37(5), 1441–1447.

Takahashi, K., Nishimura, F., Kurihara, M. et al. (2001). Subgingival microflora and antibody responses against periodontal bacteria of young Japanese patients with type 1 diabetes mellitus. *J Int Acad Periodontol*, 3(4), 104–111.

Takeuchi, K., Matsumoto, K., Furuta, M. et al. (2019). Periodontitis is associated with chronic obstructive pulmonary disease. *J Dent Res*, 98(5), 534–540.

Takeuchi, K., Ohara, T., Furuta, M., Takeshita, T. et al. (2017). Tooth loss and risk of dementia in the community: the Hisayama Study. *J Am Geriatr Soc*, 65(5), e95–e100.

Takeya, Y., Popper, J., Shimizu, Y. et al. (1984). Epidemiologic studies of coronary heart disease and stroke in Japanese men living in Japan, Hawaii and California: incidence of stroke in Japan and Hawaii. *Stroke*, 15, 15–23.

Tanaka, T., Hirano, H., Ohara, Y. et al. (2021). Oral Frailty Index-8 in the risk assessment of new-onset oral frailty and functional disability among community-dwelling older adults. *Arch Gerontol Geriatr*, 94, 104340.

Tanaka, T., Takahashi, K., Hirano, H. et al. (2018). Oral frailty as a risk factor for physical frailty and mortality in community-dwelling elderly. *J Gerontol A Biol Sci Med Sci*, 73(12), 1661–1667.

Teeuw, W.J., Gerdes, V.E., & Loos, B.G. (2010). Effect of periodontal treatment on glycemic control of diabetic patients – a systematic review and meta-analysis. *Diabetes Care*, 33(2), 421–427.

Tonetti, M.S., D'Aiuto, F., Nibali, L. et al. (2007). Treatment of periodontitis and endothelial function. *N Engl J Med*, 356(9), 911–920.

Trichopoulou, A., Kyrozis, A., Rossi, M. et al. (2015). Mediterranean diet and cognitive decline over time in an elderly Mediterranean population. *Eur J Nutr*, 54(8), 1311–1321.

Tsakos, G., Watt, R.G., Rouxel, P.L. et al. (2015). Tooth loss associated with physical and cognitive decline in older adults. *J Am Geriatr Soc*, 63(1), 91–99.

Tzeng, N.S., Chung, C.H., Yeh, C.B. et al. (2016). Are chronic periodontitis and gingivitis associated with dementia? A nationwide, retrospective, matched-cohort study in Taiwan. *Neuroepidemiology*, 47(2), 82–93.

Ueno, T., & Yurikusa, T. (2015). Effects of oral care on postoperative recovery period and state (including multidisciplinary cooperation). Role of oral care in perioperative complications in surgery. *The Current Evidence of Dental Care and Oral Health for Achieving Healthy Longevity in an Aging Society*. Japan Dental Association (Fukai K editor in chief). Japan Dental Association, 236–245.

Wakai, K., Naito, M., Naito, T. et al. (2010). Tooth loss and intakes of nutrients and foods, a nationwide survey of Japanese dentists. *Community Dent. Oral Epidemiol*, 38(1), 43–49.

Wakai, K., Naito, M., Naito, T. et al. (2013). Tooth loss and risk of hip fracture: a prospective study of male Japanese dentists. *Community Dent Oral Epidemiol*, 41(1), 48–54.

Wang, R.S., Hu, X.Y., Gu, W.J. et al. (2013). Tooth loss and risk of head and neck cancer: a meta-analysis. *PloS One*, 8(8), e71122. https://www.ncbi.nlm.nih.gov/pmc/articles/PMC3829962/pdf/pone.0079074.pdf

Watanabe, Y., Hirano, H., Arai, H. et al. (2017). Relationship between frailty and oral function in community-dwelling elderly adults. *J Am Geriatr Soc*, 65(1), 66–76.

Watt, R.G., & Sheiham, A. (2012). Integrating the common risk factor approach into a social determinants framework. *Community Dent Oral Epidemiol*, 40(4), 289–296.

Watt, R.G., Tsakos, G., de Oliveira, C., & Hamer, M. (2012). Tooth loss and cardiovascular disease mortality risk – results from the Scottish Health Survey. *PloS One*, 7(2), e30797.

World Health Organization (2010). *A Conceptual Framework for Action on the Social Determinants of Health*. Geneva: WHO. https://www.who.int/publications/i/item/9789241500852 (accessed 13 May 2024).

Xue, Q.L. (2011). The frailty syndrome: definition and natural history. *Clin Geriatr Med*, 27(1), 1–15.

Yamamoto, T., & Tsuneishi, M. (2015). Health education (including the common risk factor approach), and topical fluoride application as a measure of health education. *The Current Evidence of Dental Care and Oral Health for Achieving Healthy Longevity in an Aging Society*. Japan Dental Association (Fukai K editor in chief), 258–264.

Yamamoto, T., Kondo, K., Hirai, H. et al. (2012a). Association between self-reported dental health status and onset of dementia: a 4-year prospective cohort study of older Japanese adults from the Aichi Gerontological Evaluation Study (AGES) Project. *Psychosom Med*, 74(3), 241–248.

Yamamoto, T., Kondo, K., Misawa, J. et al. (2012b). Dental status and incident falls among older Japanese, a prospective cohort study. *BMJ Open*, 2(4).

Yamamoto, T., & Naito M. (2015). Association between oral health and main illnesses underlying conditions that necessitate long-term care: falls and fractures. *The Current Evidence of Dental Care and Oral Health for Achieving Healthy Longevity in an Aging Society*. Japan Dental Association (Fukai K editor in chief), 158–161.

Yoneyama, T., Yoshida, M., Ohrui, T. et al. (2002). Oral care reduces pneumonia in older patients in nursing homes. *J Am Geriatr Soc*, 50, 430–433.

Yoshihara, A., Watanabe, R., Nishimuta, M. et al. (2005). The relationship between dietary intake and the number of teeth in elderly Japanese subjects. *Gerodontology*, 22(4), 211–218.

Zhao, P., Xu, A., & Leung, W.K. (2022). Obesity, bone loss, and periodontitis: the interlink. *Biomolecules*, 12(7), 865.

4

Universal health coverage and effective health policy: Lessons from Japan

Oral Health for an Ageing Population: Evidence, Policy, Practice and Evaluation, First Edition. Kakuhiro Fukai.
© 2025 John Wiley & Sons Ltd. Published 2025 by John Wiley & Sons Ltd.

4.1 Introduction

Barriers to oral health services, including dental care for older people, need to be removed in order to make these vital services accessible to all. This is in line with the philosophy of universal health coverage (UHC) (WHO 2015), which is also reflected in the Sustainable Development Goals (SDGs) (UN 2015), that everyone should have access to basic health services. Oral health is a key indicator of overall health in older age. Better integration of oral healthcare into the general healthcare system is required (WHO 2020).

This chapter explains the definition and philosophy of UHC as well as how UHC achievement is assessed based on each country's circumstances and resources.

In addition, Japan is a country where dental care has been covered under the public health insurance system since 1961, and programmes for the prevention of decline in oral function are positioned within the long-term care insurance system. In addition, there is a publicly-financed system of dental health check-ups throughout infancy, childhood, adulthood and old age. Another unique aspect of Japan's approach is that measures to prevent dental diseases and oral function decline are included in national health policies such as those targeting frailty, dementia and non-communicable diseases (NCDs). For these reasons, in this chapter Japan is presented as an example of how to position dental health and dental care within an advanced, effective and stable UHC system.

4.2 Evidence-based and effective health policy

4.2.1 Evidence-based health policy

Approximately one scientific paper is published per minute in the medical field, or around 700 000 per year. Researchers' motivations range from personal and professional curiosity to career-related necessity, but they often do not have sufficient incentive to translate their research results into practice and policy-related action. The evidence that accumulates through research does not reach its full potential if it is never translated into action. It is essential for a society to establish a strong and durable cycle from research/evidence to practice and policy (Figure 4.1). The transition from evidence to practice can be achieved by drawing up clinical guidelines, establishing health promotion initiatives and enacting health policy. Putting evidence into practice in individual clinics, hospitals, institutions or communities has limited effectiveness from the standpoint of national public health.

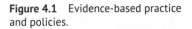

Figure 4.1 Evidence-based practice and policies.

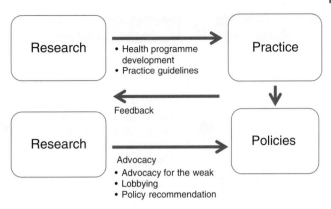

In his inverse care law, Hart (1971) noted that healthy people are more likely to access public health programmes than unhealthy people. This means that when individual healthcare professionals enact evidence-based care in the absence of a larger regional or national public health policy, they end up widening rather than narrowing the health gap (inequity in access to health care), thereby leaving the most vulnerable members of society behind. For this reason, it is essential that the process of implementing evidence-based (and data-based) practice and policy be intentionally and consistently promoted and monitored (including assessment of the effectiveness of implemented programs) at the regional and national levels.

It is essential that governments strive to implement *evidence-based* public health programmes and services, for the following two reasons, both of which stem from the basic fact that evidence-based practices are likely to be more effective than those that are not evidence-based. The first reason is that public health initiatives require great investment of financial and human resources, and these are ultimately funded by taxpayers. This means that government organizations have a vested interest in implementing programmes that are as effective as possible, not only to improve public health (which is the primary goal, of course) but also to ensure that the funding is not wasted, but instead yields a strong return on the investment. The second reason is related to ethics and human rights. Non-evidence-based public health practices have greater potential to harm the people they are intended to help, and the provision of safe and effective health services is considered to be a fundamental human right.

In order to implement and enhance the research–practice–policy cycle described earlier, there is a need to establish stronger links between researchers and policymakers. Figure 4.2 is a visualization of the pathway whereby researchers communicate their findings and policymakers gain an understanding thereof and implement the relevant policies. Researchers have little motivation to reach out to policymakers to inform them of the evidence they have found, and policymakers may lack the scientific literacy needed to translate evidence into policy, or even to understand the need for evidence-based policy. Of course, it would behove researchers to polish their communication skills and make a greater effort to transmit their findings to the public and to policymakers. And, of course, policymakers should be encouraged to improve their awareness and expertise of science. But barring such a revolution, there will, for the foreseeable future, be a great need for science writers, medical journalists, media commentators and other experts to bridge the gap between scientists and policymakers. Governments also need to establish and maintain large-scale health literacy and health education initiatives and programmes so that citizens can access high-quality, trustworthy, evidence-based health knowledge themselves.

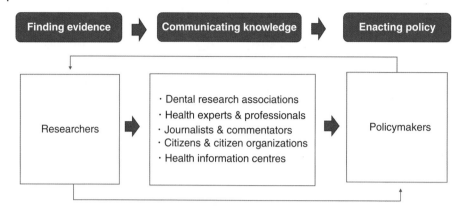

Figure 4.2 Bridging the gap between researchers and policymakers.

4.2.2 Effective health policy

Figure 4.3 shows the relationship between life expectancy and health expenditure per capita of Organisation for Economic Co-operation and Development (OECD) nations from 1995 to 2015 (OECD 2018). Although causality is unclear, a direct relationship is clearly visible: life expectancy at birth has increased along with health expenditure throughout this period for all countries shown. However, the ratio of the magnitude of increase of life expectancy with the increased cost differs among countries. These differences are largely attributable to differing healthcare systems, with the most obvious difference being the United States' reluctance to view public health as an essential responsibility of government. Increased life expectancy always requires increases in health expenditures, but a comprehensive, cost-effective,

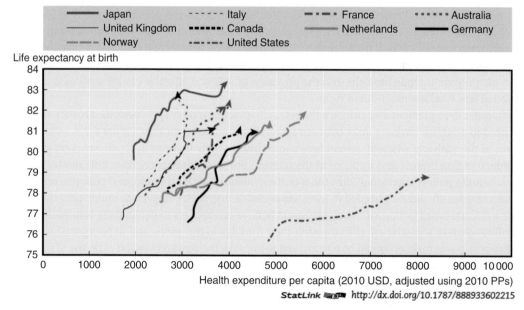

StatLink http://dx.doi.org/10.1787/888933602215

Figure 4.3 Life expectancy gains and increased health spending, selected high-income countries, 1995–2015. *Source:* OECD. Health at a Glance 2017, February 2018.

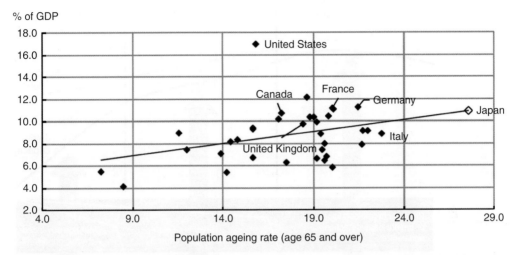

Figure 4.4 Total health expenditure and population ageing rate. *Source:* OECD Health Statics 2019/with permission of World Health Organization.

prevention-focused healthcare system can temper that increase substantially. In other words, as shown in Figure 4.4, healthcare system reform can be effective in reducing healthcare costs, particularly in an ageing society (OECD 2019).

On the other hand, oral health improvement contributes to reducing medical expenditure. Tsuneishi et al. (2017) conducted a cross-sectional study of patients aged 50–79 years using Japan's National Database of Health Insurance Claim Information and Specified Medical Checkups. The samples were 327 689, 610 087 and 654 410 eligible patients in their 50s, 60s and 70s, respectively. To describe associations between number of teeth (independent variable) and medical expenditure (primary outcome) whilst controlling for sex, they also constructed generalized linear models with a gamma distribution and log-link function by using maximum likelihood estimation. The models, which were conducted by age group, showed that medical expenditure increased by 2.4% for each tooth lost in patients in their 50s [multiplicative effect, 0.98; 95% confidence interval (CI): 0.97–0.98). The association was also found in patients in their 60s (multiplicative effect = 0.98, 95% CI: 0.98–0.99) and in those in their 70s (multiplicative effect = 0.99, 95% CI: 0.99–0.99) (Tsuneishi et al. 2017; Chávez et al. 2022).

4.2.3 Public health framework for a healthy ageing population

Biological ageing has some identifiable characteristics such as the decline of functional ability and intrinsic capacity, multimorbidity and individual diversity in old age. Figure 4.5 shows a public health framework for healthy ageing, published by WHO (2015). Numerous intervention points can be identified for actions to promote healthy ageing and foster functional ability. This can be achieved in two ways: (1) by supporting the building and maintenance of intrinsic capacity; and (2) by enabling those with a decline in their functional capacity to do the things that are important to them.

These general trajectories can be divided into three stages: (1) a period of relatively high and stable capacity; (2) a period of declining capacity; and (3) a period of significant loss of capacity. To intervene in each of these stages, we can take many actions such as establishing universal medical

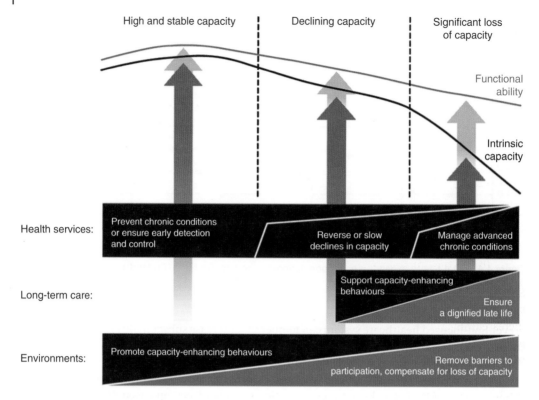

Figure 4.5 A public health framework for healthy ageing: opportunities for public health action across the life course. *Source:* WHO (2015b).

care and a long-term care system in each country in addition to providing a healthy environment. For example, early care to reduce declines in capacities might include family and community members encouraging older people to become more active and assisting them with doing so. Another example is encouraging older people to eat well. These interventions can be implemented more easily if the older person lives in an enabling environment.

This strategy is designed to encourage a fundamental paradigm shift in the way health services are funded, managed and delivered so that all people have access to health services that respond to their preferences, are coordinated around their needs and are safe, effective, timely, efficient and of an acceptable quality.

One important characteristic of ageing is individual diversity. Some people maintain the level of oral functional ability required for daily living throughout their lives, but others experience a decline in functional ability and fall below the disability threshold at some point in their life. In order to prevent oral function decline in older people, oral health conditions should be maintained through preventive care and public health actions.

From the perspective of prevention and health promotion, it is considered more effective to implement oral health promotion programmes before the occurrence of oral health problems and functional decline in independent older people. Therefore, it is important to implement screening programmes in community settings. To this end, public health programmes for prevention of oral function decline can be integrated within prevention-focused general health programs.

4.3 The global challenge of UHC

4.3.1 UHC for older persons

4.3.1.1 What is UHC?

Universal health coverage means that all people in a society have access to the health services they need, when and where they need them, without financial hardship. This includes the full range of essential health services: health promotion, prevention, treatment, rehabilitation, and palliative care. It is safe to say that no country can ever meet all of these conditions perfectly; however, establishing this as a clear national and/or global objective is essential from a human rights and health equity standpoint. The World Health Organization (WHO) defines UHC as follows:

> UHC means that all individuals and communities receive the health services they need without suffering financial hardship. It includes the full spectrum of essential, quality health services, from health promotion to prevention, treatment, rehabilitation, and palliative care across the life course.

Since the WHO published its 2010 report on financing world health systems, entitled 'Health systems financing: the path to universal coverage', international awareness of this concept has increased. Since 2008, the United Nations General Assembly has adopted a resolution each year on a different theme related to global health and foreign policy. As part of that series, in 2012 a resolution on UHC was adopted, formalizing its importance to the world health community.

4.3.1.2 The three dimensions and two components of the WHO's UHC report

According to the WHO, UHC consists of three dimensions: the range of health services provided, the funding of those services, and the percentage of the population covered. This concept, known as the 'coverage cube', is shown in Figure 4.6. The ideal, of course, is to provide all services

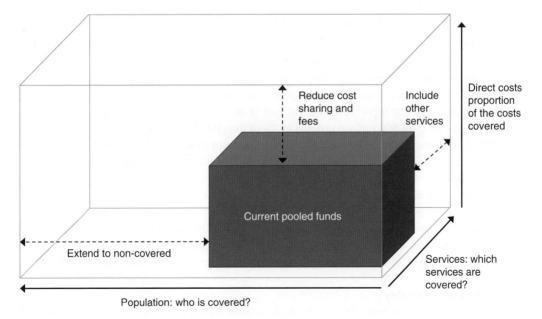

Figure 4.6   The three dimensions of UHC. *Source:* WHO (2015).

completely free to all people. Individual nations, however, have limited resources, and each country may have different priorities and preferences. Governments must therefore decide how to expand coverage along these three dimensions (Maeda 2014; WHO 2017).

4.3.2 Access to dental care for older adults

Regarding access to dental care, we must first be clear about what sort of care people should have access to. Harris (2013) defined access to dental care as the state in which both individuals and communities can obtain preventive care, relief of symptoms and restorative care. It would also be appropriate to add consultation and education to that list.

Next, we need to look closely at the factors that either facilitate or prevent access to dental care. Based on the WHO's UHC Cube, the 2023 World Dental Federation white paper (FDI 2023) identifies three core factors: availability, affordability and acceptability. Availability refers to whether or not an adequate number of dental clinics (and the accompanying human and material resources) exists in a certain location, and how easy it is for older residents to get there (including both distance and means of transportation). Affordability refers to the cost of services and is also heavily influenced by the healthcare system and related insurance systems. Acceptability is related to health literacy and individual preferences as well as cultural and social barriers such as language and communication issues. Of particular concern with older patients is that they often lose motivation to continue routine preventive maintenance, and this might be due to either anxiety or apathy. Aida et al. (2022) cites McLaughlin and Wyszewianski (2002) in proposing an additional core factor of dental care access for older adults: accommodation. This refers to the extent to which dental care providers and institutions make specific adjustments and arrangements to improve accessibility for older and disabled patients, such as updating to barrier-free facilities, visiting nursing homes and conducting home visits.

Improving access to dental care starts with identifying which of these factors need to be improved, implementing specific interventions, and then assessing the effectiveness thereof.

4.3.3 How does the WHO monitor progress towards UHC?

In 2017, the WHO and the World Bank published a global report tracking the progress of UHC (WHO 2017). This report investigated the number of people globally who cannot access essential health services as well as how many fall into poverty due to lack of health care access (related to SDG indicator 1.1.1) or due to spending too high a proportion of their budget on healthcare expenses (SDG indicator 3.8.2). The report revealed that half of the world's people do not receive the health services they need. Over 800 million people (11.7% of the global population) are forced to allocate over 10% of their household budget to healthcare expenses, and about 100 million people (1.4% of the global population) fall into extreme poverty as a result of health expenditures.

Progress towards UHC is a continual process that is sensitive to shifting demographics, epidemiological trends and the expectations of the local populace. The goal of UHC monitoring activities is to encourage governments to make progress towards ensuring that people in need of educational, preventive, treatment-oriented, rehabilitative or end-of-life health services receive them, and also that such services are of sufficient quality to realize significant individual and public health improvement. The levels of service coverage vary widely between countries (WHO 2017, 2021c, 2022).

4.3.3.1 UHC and inequality

The degree of coverage of essential health services (defined as the average coverage of essential services based on tracer interventions that include reproductive, maternal, newborn and child health, infectious diseases, NCDs and service capacity and access, among the general and the

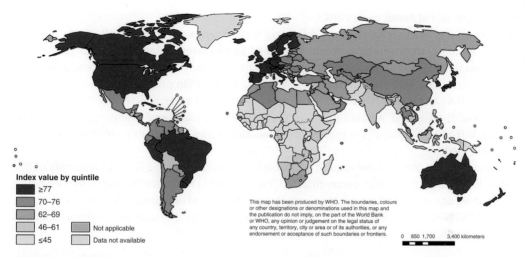

Figure 4.7 UHC service coverage index by country, 2015: SDG indicator 3.8.1. *Source:* WHO (2017).

most disadvantaged populations) of a country can be measured and reported via the UHC Service Coverage Index. This index is quantified via a unitless scale of 0–100, which is computed as the geometric mean of 14 tracer indicators of health service coverage. The tracer indicators are as follows, organized by four components of service coverage: (1) reproductive, maternal, newborn and child health; (2) infectious diseases; (3) NCDs; and (4) service capacity and access. There are not yet enough data to correlate the UHC service coverage index with key dimensions of inequality. In the meantime, service coverage inequalities can be ascertained by looking at narrower service coverage indicators such as maternal and child health services. For a set of seven basic services related to mother and child health, only 17% of mothers and infants in the lowest wealth quintile in low- and lower-middle-income countries were able to access at least six of the seven services, compared with 74% of those in the highest wealth quintile (2005–2015 data) (WHO 2017) (Figure 4.7).

4.3.3.2 UHC and financial hardship

Families frequently experience financial difficulty due to healthcare-related expenses. The WHO divides such financial difficulty into two levels: 'catastrophic spending on health', which is non-reimbursed spending that exceeds the household's ability to pay; and 'impoverishing spending on health', which means a household has to shift finances from non-medical budget categories, such as food, housing and clothing in order to pay for health services, to the point that the budget allocated for those categories falls below the poverty line [Global Burden of Disease Study (GBD) UHC Collaborators 2019].

4.3.4 UHC, SDGs and oral health

In 2015, the United Nations adopted a new development agenda entitled, *Transforming Our World: The 2030 Agenda for Sustainable Development.* This report laid out 17 SDGs, where health is prominently positioned as goal 3 (SDG 3). SDG 3 includes 13 targets covering all major health priorities. The 2030 Agenda differs from the Millennium Development Goal agenda, which was in effect from 2000 to 2015, in that the newer agenda incorporates the implementation of health monitoring goals at the global, regional and national levels (Kieny 2017).

4.3.4.1 The role of dental care in UHC

Oral health has been included in the following WHO resolutions: WHA60.17 (2007) ('On oral health: Action plan for promotion and integrated disease prevention'), WHA69.3 (2016) ('On the global strategy and action plan on ageing and health 2016–2020: Towards a world in which everyone can live a long and healthy life'), WHA72.2 (2019) ('On primary health care; and decisions'), WHA72(11) (2019) ('On the follow-up to the political declaration of the third high-level meeting of the General Assembly on the prevention and control of non-communicable diseases'), WHA73(12) (2020) ('On the decade of healthy ageing 2020–2030') and WHA74.5 (2021) ('On oral health').

In addition, the 'Political declaration of the high-level meeting of the General Assembly on the prevention and control of non-communicable diseases' (2011) recognized that oral diseases pose a major challenge and called for common responses to NCDs and oral disease (UN 2011).

WHA73(7) (2020) and WHA74.5 (2021) included a commitment to strengthen efforts to address oral health within the framework of UHC (WHO 2020, 2021d).

4.3.5 Achieving healthy longevity by implementing UHC

As we face the rapid ageing of our population, which is proceeding at a rate never before experienced by humankind, many efforts to deal with this problem have been initiated in various fields of academic research as well as in medical, health, welfare and community settings. In order to realize a society where elderly people can live their lives in peace and with dignity, it is essential to develop health and medical care systems that provide high-quality healthcare services.

It is inevitable that in old age, people experience a decline in the functions of daily living and become more susceptible to diseases. The ageing of the population is a result of decreasing mortality in adulthood and old age, as well as in the neonatal period and early childhood, which has been achieved by acquiring knowledge, accumulating scientific evidence and developing advanced technologies. However, population ageing has also extended the period during which people require care, and this will continue to increase the healthcare investment needed at the national and community level.

Under the present circumstances, providing sufficient healthcare to all elderly individuals requires adequate human and social resources, a social security system which includes a healthcare system and rests on a solid financial foundation, and the accumulation of scientific evidence. Moreover, it will be necessary to inform the citizenry, policymakers and healthcare workers regarding the outcomes of the various measures. Another important political issue is how to extend the healthy period during old age.

Furthermore, dental and oral health is an essential element for the maintenance of quality of life (QOL) throughout one's life. Research has also made it clear that dental and oral health contribute to the maintenance and improvement of systemic health status. Therefore, it is essential that we develop a social system that allows everyone to receive high-quality dental care and oral health services even during old age.

In addition, collaboration between the medical and dental fields, and between professionals in both fields, towards the development of a more effective system of healthcare provision is needed. To this end, it is necessary to accumulate clearer evidence and take specific actions in order to situate dental care and oral health firmly within the social security system and healthcare policy, which in turn will facilitate the contribution of dental care to the realization of healthy longevity.

STEP 1 Needs assessment and monitoring	STEP 2 Determining the appropriate healthcare system and provisions	STEP 3 Reducing the global burden of oral diseases and disability based on human rights	STEP 4 Contributing to and achieving a healthy ageing society
1. Determine the core oral health indicator and assess the oral healthcare needs 2. Data collection of health manpower and oral healthcare system 3. Continuous data collection and sharing	1. Provide policymakers with evidence regarding policy effectiveness 2. Inter-professional and cross-sector collaboration for a sustainable system, such as the common risk factor approach of NCDs 3. Increasing people's awareness of oral health measures and the value of oral health 4. Improving oral healthcare outreach via integrated oral/general healthcare system	1. Evidence-based oral health programme 2. Prevention/control of tooth loss and oral diseases 3. Reducing oral health risk factors for NCDs and frailty 4. Contribute to closing the health inequality gap 5. Strengthen health policy	1. Shared values of general/oral health 2. Active ageing in a healthy community 3. Seeking a more effective/efficient healthcare system 4. Continue monitoring health inequality

Figure 4.8 Four steps for achieving oral health in an ageing society. *Source:* Fukai K et al. 2017/FDI World Dental Federation.

The ageing of populations worldwide is rapidly accelerating. However, the global burden of oral disease remains a critical and often underestimated problem. As ageing progresses globally, oral health maintenance becomes a matter not only of public health, but also of human rights. Therefore, in low- and middle-income countries, policymakers are seeking to realize UHC, including oral health, even as they struggle with severe resource limitations.

To achieve and maintain global oral health, I have proposed an ongoing global monitoring cycle consisting of the following four steps: needs assessment, implementation of appropriate healthcare systems and provisions, reducing the global burden of oral disease, and working to achieve a healthy ageing society (Fukai et al. 2017) (Figure 4.8).

Rather than a unidirectional information flow from high-income to low- and middle-income countries, the proposed system would establish a multidirectional information-sharing cycle that would benefit all countries. To make this possible, however, we must develop a standardized set of core oral health indicators that all countries use, as well as a global repository for gathering, compiling and sharing the data.

This system would allow each country to move forward at its own pace and in locally appropriate ways, making it more effective and efficient in the long run than the current pattern of setting unrealistic goals that all countries are expected to achieve by a certain point in time.

4.4 Japan's public healthcare system

4.4.1 Challenges faced by Japan in a super-ageing society

The current Japanese life expectancy is 81.3 in males and 87.3 in females, making Japan the current global leader in longevity [Ministry of Health, Labour and Welfare (MHLW) of Japan 2022b]. The survival rates of males and females at 75 years of age are 75.6% and 88.1%, respectively (MHLW of Japan 2022b). At 90 years of age, the survival rates are 26.5% in males and 50.5% in females. This means that over half of Japanese females live past the age of 90. On the other hand, it is an unavoidable biological reality that ageing causes increased vulnerability to disease and disability. Therefore, the current challenge for Japan, at both the individual and policymaking levels, is to shift the focus from longevity to 'healthy longevity'. A number of methods for measuring healthy longevity have been proposed and developed by various researchers and organizations around the world. In Japan, healthy longevity is defined as a lack of limitation on activities of daily living (ADLs), and it is measured subjectively via questionnaire. The percentage of those perceiving limitations on their ADLs is 30% at age 75 and 50% at age (MHLW of Japan 2019). The incidence of dementia increases rapidly above the age of 75, with 80% of those above age 95 being diagnosed as having dementia.

Fortunately, Japan was able to establish a UHC system as early as 1961, and it also launched its publicly funded long-term care system in 2001. Thanks to these initiatives, all Japanese people have a basic level of access to medical, dental and long-term care in their old age. However, the combination of rapid ageing and a comprehensive publicly funded healthcare system has resulted in an increasingly untenable financial burden on the government.

From the viewpoint of the Japanese national budget, during the past three decades, the cost of the social security system has tripled from JPY11.6 trillion in 1990 to 34.4 trillion in 2019 (National Institute of Population and Social Security Research 2021) (Figure 4.9). However, the applicable revenue has remained unchanged during this time, so the entirety of the increased cost has directly contributed to the increasing national debt. Due in part to this, the current debt of Japan is higher than it has been at any time since the end of World War II.

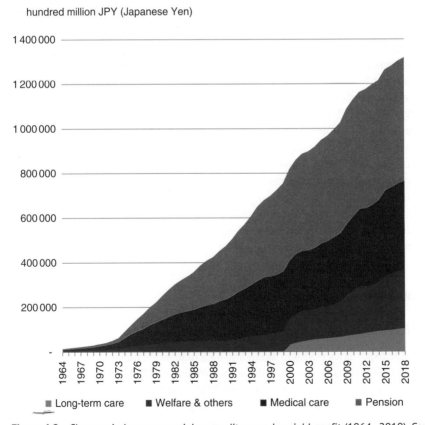

hundred million JPY (Japanese Yen)

■ Long-term care　■ Welfare & others　■ Medical care　■ Pension

Figure 4.9 Changes in Japanese social expenditure and social benefit (1964–2019). *Source:* Adapted from The National Institute of Population and Social Security Research 2021.

4.4.2   Japan's current health policy framework for a sustainable social security system

Sixty per cent of deaths in Japan are caused by NCDs such as cancer, cardiovascular disease, cerebrovascular disease and pneumonia, and these diseases account for 30% of all medical expenditure (MHLW of Japan 2022c). In addition, NCDs such as cerebrovascular disease cause 30% of long-term care dependency, and if dementia, frailty and falls are added, that percentage rises to more than 80% (MHLW of Japan 2022b). Therefore, prevention and control of these diseases is considered essential to increase HLE.

The current goals of Japanese government health policy, as well as for healthcare professionals themselves, are: (1) to prevent and control NCDs, and (2) to prevent frailty and thereby reduce dependency on long-term care.

To achieve these goals, Japan has already established high-quality medical infrastructure and care that is vertically oriented, usually proceeding from local to regional to national-level institutions. However, more recently, government policy has resulted in a concerted effort to develop a disease-specific (cancer, cerebrovascular and cardiovascular diseases, dementia, diabetes and pulmonary diseases), horizontally integrated (multi-sectoral) medical care system, and this system expressly includes dental care. This horizontal system has developed in tandem with an evidence-based paradigm shift whereby oral health is now seen as playing an essential role in overall physical and mental health.

Another type of infrastructure being developed to address these two goals (preventing NCDs and preventing frailty and dependency) is an integrated community care system. This system is designed to bring together a network of medical and long-term care providers to form an integrated and prevention-focused healthcare system that is age-friendly and locally oriented, so that elderly users can obtain these services without travelling long distances to large institutions. By integrating the medical care and long-term care services, this system is also designed to eliminate redundancies and thereby reduce costs (Fukai 2019) (Figure 4.10).

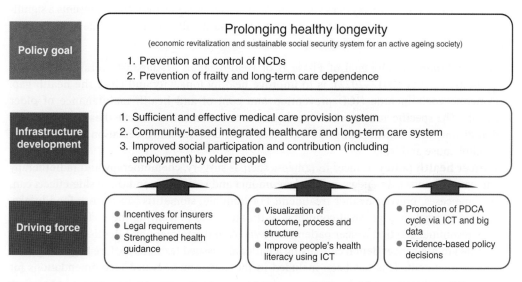

Figure 4.10   Japan's current health policy framework for a sustainable social security system. ICT: information and communications technology; PDCA: plan–do–check–act.

4.4.3   How oral health and cooperative medical and dental care contribute to healthy longevity

Although the oral health status of the Japanese people has improved during the past three decades, oral disease remains prevalent and the oral health gap persists. However, in order to forge ahead towards effective and sustainable solutions to these challenges, we must think beyond the narrow confines of the oral health field and set our sights on truly multi-sectoral collaboration, specifically including improved medical and dental care cooperation.

This recommendation is based on accumulated evidence from the past two decades suggesting that several pathways connect dental care and oral health with HLE: (1) age-related changes and ageing; (2) life expectancy; (3) NCDs as the main causes of death and the common risk factors thereof; (4) diseases that cause conditions requiring long-term care; (5) health promotion activities such as nutrition, exercise and rest; and (6) socioeconomic factors.

Based on this body of scientific evidence, a 'one health approach', which reorients oral healthcare as an integral component of general health policy, would be an effective way to decrease the National Health Insurance (NHI) budget while preventing NCDs and frailty and achieving further improvements in oral health. Health policymakers should recognize the great and often overlooked potential of oral health to contribute to a sustainable social security system. These challenges would contribute to global health and sustainable development.

In the context of Japanese health policy, the importance of oral health was accorded greater recognition in 2011, when the Dental and Oral Health Promotion Act was established. Article 1 of this act included the statement, 'oral health plays an absolutely necessary role in achieving individual health and well-being'.

Although the main role of dental professionals remains the prevention and control of dental disease to prevent the decline of oral function, recently implemented evidence-based health policies have shifted towards seeing dental care as an important contributing factor in general health, particularly in areas such as NCD and frailty/dependency prevention. This portends a meaningful expansion of the role of dental clinics in the context of the larger healthcare system. The following is a list of current and planned nationally funded programmes that expressly recommend the linking of dental and oral health services with general medical services (this trend represents a significant step towards translating evidence into practice and it calls for a large-scale shift towards multi-sectoral and interprofessional cooperation):

1) **Health Japan 21**. The goal of Phase II of Health Japan 21, Japan's overarching health promotion policy (2013–2022), is to improve healthy longevity and close the health gap. Concrete goals include NCD prevention and control and health maintenance of older people. The specific activities and behaviours recommended to achieve these goals include dental and oral health alongside exercise, nutrition, smoking cessation, avoidance of alcohol abuse and rest.

2) **Cancer health policy**. Cancer treatments such as surgery, chemotherapy and radiotherapy can cause serious side-effects such as pneumonia and stomatitis, and these side-effects can, in some cases, prevent further treatment. For example, stomatitis can disturb food intake, leading to weakened physical condition. With an eye to preventing these side-effects, it is now recommended that cancer patients undergo dental treatment by a dentist who has been certified in pre-cancer dental care (using a nationally issued textbook) before beginning their cancer treatment. This has been included in the government-issued recommendations for cancer specialists since 2013.

3) **Dementia policy**. In the dementia policy paper called the 'New Orange Plan' (2015–2025) and also in the national dementia policy outline established in 2019, it is clearly stated that community-based dental care plays a role in early diagnosis and prevention of cognitive decline and dementia. In addition, the first ever government-issued set of dental care guidelines for older people with dementia was published in 2019.

4) **Diabetes policy**. The national policy for the prevention and control of diabetic nephropathy (an NCD) has included an oral health programme designed to control periodontal disease and improve eating behaviour since 2016. Also in 2016, a chapter on the relationship between diabetes and periodontitis was included in the Japanese Clinical Practice Guideline for Diabetes (for medical specialists). The evidence level of this relationship was raised again in 2019.

5) **Prevention of frailty**. The importance of frailty prevention was explicitly stated in the national guidelines for elderly health promotion. Prevention of oral functional decline has been included a key factor in this document since 2018. In addition, in 2016, dental clinics began offering nationally funded dental check-ups and health guidance for elderly people aged 75 and older. This programme aims not only to prevent decline in oral health and function but also to prevent frailty and reduce dependence on long-term care.

6) **Prevention and control of metabolic syndrome**. A national system of specific health check-ups and health guidance for the prevention of metabolic syndrome, which targets people over 40 years old, was implemented in April 2008. As part of this system, health education materials designed to prevent metabolic syndrome (diabetes, obesity, and heart disease), as well as related risk factors such as periodontal disease and chewing function decline, have been developed. This national system of specific health check-ups and specific health guidance is reviewed and updated once every 5 years. In 2018, question items regarding subjective chewing function were added because a decline in chewing function is indicative of dental disease and tooth loss.

4.4.4 Japan's public health system and UHC system: a brief history

In 2016, under the banner, 'no one will be left behind', the UN adopted a set of 17 SDGs to be achieved by 2030. Goal 3 focused on ensuring health and well-being for all humans at all stages of life. Of the nine specific sub-goals within goal 3, two were newly included: (1) reducing premature death via NCD prevention and control and (2) achieving universal health coverage. As governments all over the world work to implement universal health coverage, there is a common misperception that this primarily entails developing a country's medical care insurance system (increasing the number of people or diseases covered). However, this focus often turns out to be short-sighted and end in failure. One reason is that governments quickly run into financial constraints, causing them to abandon the goal altogether. Or they succeed in increasing coverage for certain diseases or for certain segments of society, effectively increasing the health gap rather than narrowing it. Rather than focusing exclusively on the medical care insurance system, what is needed is a more consistent and all-encompassing approach to public health. The experience of Japan shows how this approach can be successful over the long term (Reich et al. 2011).

An outside observer may be tempted to credit this accomplishment to Japan's post-war 'economic miracle' and UHC, but the story is more complicated than that and it starts much earlier, as far back as the Meiji period or even before.

At the beginning of the 20th century, Japan was already busy establishing a strong education system that would improve the literacy rate. Healthy eating habits and other daily routines, such as taking baths and exercising, certainly played a part. However, it was the public health efforts led by midwives, public health nurses and school health nurses in the 1940s and 1950s that really

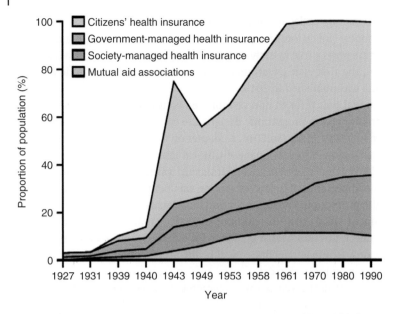

Figure 4.11 Trends in health insurance coverage in Japan, 1927–1990. *Source:* Ikegami N et al 2011/ with permission of Elsevier.

started putting downward pressure on the neonatal mortality rate. Community-based midwives rode their bicycles to homes to provide professional assistance with childhood at very low rates and often for free. Public health nurses also travelled to individual homes and contributed to health literacy and community sanitation efforts. School health initiatives brought nurses, dentists and doctors into the schools to engage in health education and promotion initiatives.

All of these wheels started turning decades before universal health coverage was achieved. In fact, as seen in Figure 4.11, the implementation of UHC was itself an extremely long and gradual process, beginning with the passage of the Health Insurance Act for company employees in 1922 and making another leap forward with volunteer, community-based local government initiatives to provide 'citizens' health insurance' in agricultural-oriented communities in the 1930s. It was due to these efforts that by 1943, 70% of the Japanese population was already covered under some form of health insurance. Finally, in 1958, the national government enacted and funded a comprehensive citizen's health insurance system that notably included mandatory enrolment and, over the next 3 years (1961), brought the total number of people covered up to 100% of the population (Ikegami et al. 2011). The purpose of this brief history is to emphasize the fact that Japan's success in this area was at least 40 years in the making and was rooted in education and community-level public health efforts. It is evident, therefore, that a sudden attempt to create a national-level UHC system is likely to end in failure, or at least disillusionment.

4.4.5 The medical care insurance system in Japan

As outlined in the previous section, the history of medical care insurance in Japan began with the passing of the Health Insurance Act in 1922. Thereafter, coverage was gradually extended by way of the National Health Insurance Act of 1938 and the various mutual aid association acts established from the 1950s to the beginning of the 1960s. Universal coverage under a public medical care insurance system was achieved in 1961 with the amendment of the National Health Insurance Act (Ikegami 2014) (Figure 4.12):

- Expenditures for health insurance are financed through insurance premiums (50%) and public funds (state subsidy 26%, local subsidy 13%).
- Japan's system for the remuneration of medical services is based on the fee-for-service format and free access.
- Care can be accessed via medical care facilities such as hospitals (public < 20%, private > 80%) and clinics (public < 5%, private > 95%)

Figure 4.13 shows coverage of dental care by the NHI system (MHLW of Japan 2022d). In Japan, most dental treatment is covered by the public health insurance system, as illustrated in

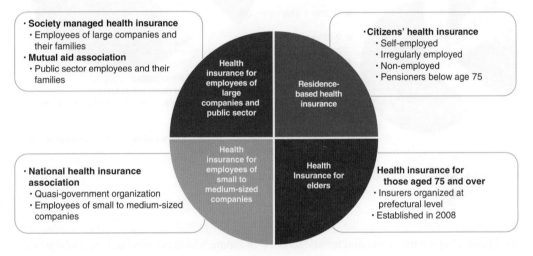

Figure 4.12 Health insurance programmes in Japan. *Source:* Ikegami (2014).

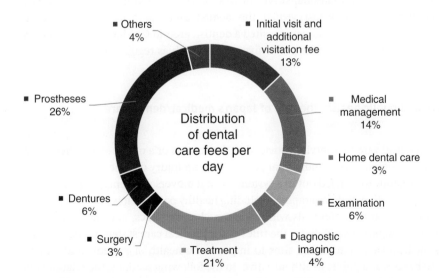

Figure 4.13 Coverage of dental care by National Health Insurance system. *Source:* Adapted from MHLW of Japan (2021) Vital Statistics of Japan.

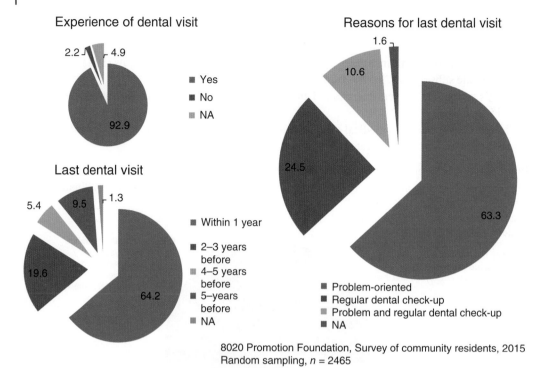

Figure 4.14 shows the results of a national survey of 2465 Japanese community residents. The figure shows when the participants last visited the dentist and the reason for that visit. Approximately 2% of the respondents had never visited a dentist, around 60% had visited a dentist in the past year, and around 35% visited for preventive reasons such as regular check-ups (Fukai et al. 2014).

4.4.6 Dental care and public health: the role of Japan's medical/dental care fee schedule

We usually think of medical care as a service provided in the context of a one-to-one relationship between a medical professional and an individual patient with an injury or illness. Public health initiatives, on the other hand, are carried out in a systematic and universal manner, provided to all people in a particular population or demographic, including healthy people. However, as a population is defined as a collection of individuals with common characteristics, and medical care is provided systematically and universally under the rules of the medical care system in the country, a universal-access medical care system that aims to improve the health of patients and patient populations can also be seen as a public health initiative. In the following sections, the relationship between medical and dental care and public health is discussed, with particular consideration given to the role of the medical/dental care fee system in Japan.

Figure 4.14 Visits to the dentist by Japanese community residents.

the figure. This is a unique characteristic of UHC in Japan, which is found in very few countries in the world.

4.4.7 Japan's National Health Insurance system

Since 1961, Japan has provided medical care to all citizens under a publicly funded NHI system. Characteristics of the system are as follows:

1) Patients can freely visit any clinic or hospital in the country.
2) Fees are charged on a per-action basis (each action, such as an examination, a test, a diagnosis, a prescription or a treatment, is assigned a separate fee)
3) Medical/dental practitioners are free to open clinics or hospitals anywhere at any time.

Medical care covered under the insurance system can be provided only by medical professionals (doctors, dentists and pharmacists) who are registered with the MHLW in accordance with the Health Insurance Act. Once registered in the system, medical professionals must practise in accordance with the detailed medical treatment procedures and rules set by the MHLW. Therefore, even though more than 99% of dental clinics are privately owned institutions, most of them must operate in accordance with the detailed national regulations in order to be covered under the NHI system.

Japan's NHI system is funded by a combination of insurance premiums (paid by all residents), the government (taxpayer-funded, including local, regional and national sources) and patients themselves (out-of-pocket payments at time of treatment – usually 30% of the cost). National government expenditure accounts for approximately 25% of all medical expenses (around JPY10 trillion, which is 10% of the national budget). However, when the government determines the annual budget for the next fiscal year, it has the authority to revise the medical fee compensation system in accordance with changes in the overall national budget. This means that the government does have mechanisms whereby it can control burden of medical expenditures on the national budget. This is important because the national financial burden of the health insurance system is constantly increasing due to advancements in medical technology and the increasing elderly population (who are at greater risk of illness and injury).

4.4.8 How the medical fee system works

The national medical fee schedule determines the unit price of each individual medical action (examination, diagnosis, prescription, treatment, etc.), and the fee schedule has an outsized impact on the nation's medical expenditures as a whole. The medical fee system is usually revised once every 2 years. The purpose of these regular revisions is: (1) coverage for new treatments and technologies; (2) reduction of expenditures for existing medical practices deemed unnecessary or less desirable from an evidence-based public health standpoint; (3) realization of policy goals; and (4) reduction of disparities between medical institutions. The revision of medical fees is carried out through two steps: (1) determining the overall budget goal for the upcoming 2-year period; and (2) determining the unit fees for various medical actions as well as drug prices.

Once every 2 years the overall medical expenditure budget for the fiscal year beginning in April is determined by the Cabinet and announced by the end of December of the previous year as part of the overall budget allocation process. In determining the medical expenditure budget, the Cabinet refers to the medical fee revisions proposed by the Medical Affairs Bureau of the Social Security Council, an advisory body to the MHLW, and the Medical Insurance Subcommittee of the MHLW's Insurance Bureau.

The next step in the process of revising the medical fee structure, which is completed by March, is to revise the fees of individual medical actions and drug prices. This is carried out by the Insurance Bureau of the MHLW based on a report drawn up and submitted by the Central Medical Insurance Medical Care Council at the ministry's request. The council members include representatives from the major insurers, medical care providers and public interest representatives, but the ministry's Insurance Bureau itself exercises great influence over the final determinations.

Fee revisions are applied mainly to medical actions, because drug prices and material prices are determined largely by market forces. The percentage of overall fees accounted for by medical actions varies greatly by profession. For example, 80% of medical care fees and 90% of dental care fees are accounted for by medical actions, while only 20% of pharmacy fees are accounted for by medical actions (the ratio is therefore 1:1.2:0.3).

Once the budget revisions are determined, the revised medical fees are calculated by applying a percentage increase or decrease to the previous year's fees. For example, the 2018 revision of medical fees resulted in dental care fees being increased by 0.69% compared with the previous year. This amounts to an overall increase of over 20 billion yen. These fees largely correspond to increased personnel expenses due to increasing numbers of patients and medical actions, along with increasing fees for medical actions.

4.4.9 Medical fee revisions as the bridge between medical/dental care and public health

The end goal of both medical care and public health is individual and societal health and well-being. The NHI system, which covers both medical care and long-term nursing care, is the central pillar of a nation's public health policies, programmes and expenditures. In the policy guidelines for the 2020 medical fee revisions (MHLW of Japan, 2019b), far more dental care-related measures were included than in previous years. Examples include: (1) inclusion of dental-related measures in regional comprehensive care objectives; (2) promotion of home medical care which includes dental care; (3) multidisciplinary cooperation between medical and dental professionals; (4) prevention and control of severe oral diseases, prevention of oral function decline, and improvement of oral function; and (5) promotion of continuous oral health maintenance by supporting and enhancing the role of family and community-based dentists. All of these are public health priorities that are influencing and expanding the priorities of dental care. This illustrates the importance of pursuing synergistic, interdisciplinary collaboration between these two fields.

Raising dental treatment fees would be the easiest way to improve the quality of dental care provided to the population. However, based on the demographic composition of the population, the current economic circumstances and the state of government financial resources in Japan, it is unlikely that dental fees can be substantially increased in the future. Instead, the most effective approach to improving the quality of dental and oral care is to recognize that the prevalence of dental diseases is still higher than other diseases and that quality dental care is still not reaching those who need it the most. The oral health gap remains.

The growing preponderance of evidence showing the link between oral health and general health (see Chapter 3 for a comprehensive review) signals the need for a completely new framework of practice and policy incorporating medical and dental collaboration. Dental/oral health is now positioned as an essential element in all areas of health policy, including NCDs and frailty prevention, and this requires large-scale multi-sectoral and interprofessional cooperation. Therefore, public health and dental care services must be integrated under a single medical fee system.

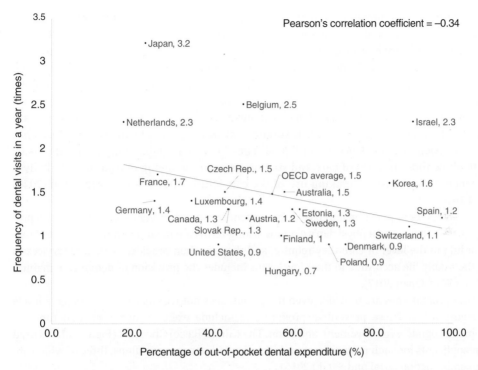

Figure 4.15 The association between the percentage of out-of-pocket dental expenditures and the average annual number of dental visits per patient in the OECD countries in 2011, or the nearest year for which data were available. *Source:* Aida J et al. 2020/with permission of Elsevier.

Most dental treatment in Japan is covered by NHI, which is funded by a combination of taxes, individual insurance premiums, and out-of-pocket payments. Around 99% of dental care facilities are private, while only 0.39% are public. Private clinics must follow government guidelines.

Around 50% of Japanese people visit dental clinics every year, where integrated dental treatment, including prevention of oral disease, is provided (8020 Promotion Foundation 2015; Aida et al. 2020) (Figures 4.14 and 4.15). Some prevention programmes, such as mother and child health, school health and elderly health, are provided to community residents (Zaitsu et al. 2018).

Elderly patients over 75 tend to stop visiting dental clinics, so there is a great need to implement in-hospital and home dental care provision. However, provision of dental care alone cannot close the oral health gap. Advanced community oral health programmes and multi-sectoral collaboration are needed.

4.4.10 Long-term care insurance in Japan

A significant decline in physical and mental capacity can limit an older person's ability to be self-sufficient and participate in society. While rehabilitation, assistive technology and access to a supportive and inclusive environment can improve the situation, many people at some point in their lives will no longer be able to do things for themselves without support and assistance. Access to high-quality, long-term care is essential for such people to maintain their functional capacity, enjoy their basic human rights and live with dignity.

Previous approaches to providing long-term care have relied heavily on informal carers, mainly family members and particularly women, who often did not receive the necessary training and support, such as care leave or insurance. Informal carers often experience a severe burden that affects their physical and mental health. Furthermore, this inequitable model of care is becoming unsustainable as the proportion of older people (many of whom have no family) increases and the proportion of younger people who can provide care decreases.

In response to these challenges, Japan established a publicly funded, long-term care insurance system. The Long-Term Care Insurance Act was approved by the Diet in December 1997 and has been in effect since 1 April 2000. The objective of public long-term care insurance is to allow those in need of care and support as result of ageing to lead their daily lives as independently as possible, making use of the capabilities they possess (Aida et al. 2020) (Figure 4.16).

The procedures for application and use of this system are shown in Figure 4.17. Based on a preliminary questionnaire and a physician's diagnosis, long-term care insurance applicants are classified according to the level of care they require, and they are then provided with care services to support their daily life according to their level. This includes the provision of dental care maintenance (MHLW of Japan 2017).

Preventive programmes are provided even if a person does not require care services (care levels 1–5 in Figure 4.17). These preventive programmes include exercise, nutrition, oral function improvement, cognitive improvement, and so on. The Kihon (Basic) Checklist (Figure 4.18) is used to screen applicants for such programmes and includes 25 interview questions, three of which are related to oral function (Arai and Sataki 2015).

The public long-term care insurance system is financed by premiums paid by individual users as well as government subsidies.

Decade	Elderly population %		Major policies
1960s Beginning of welfare policies for the elderly	5.7% (1960)	1963	Act on Social Welfare Service for Elderly passed ◇ Intensive care homes for the elderly created ◇ Legislation on home helpers for the elderly
1970s Expansion of healthcare expenditures for the elderly	7.1% (1970)	1973	Free healthcare for the elderly
1980s Social hospitalization and bedridden elderly become social problems	9.1% (1980)	1982 1989	Passage of the Health and Medical Service Act for the Aged ◇ Adoption of payment of copayments for elderly healthcare, etc. Establishment of the Plan (10-year strategy for the promotion of health and welfare for the elderly) ◇ Promotion of urgent preparation of facilities and in-home welfare services
1990s Promotion of the Gold Plan	12.0% (1990)	1994	Establishment of the New Gold Plan (new 10-year strategy for the promotion of health and welfare for the elderly) ◇ Improvement of in-home long-term care
Preparation for adoption of long-term care insurance system	14.5% (1995)	1996 1997	Policy agreement by the three coalition parties Coalition party agreement on creation of a long-term care insurance system Passage of Long-Term Care Insurance Act
2000s Implementation of long-term care insurance system	17.3% (2000)	2000 2005	Implementation of long-term care insurance Partial revision of the Long-Term Care Insurance Act

Figure 4.16 Japan's welfare policies for the elderly over five decades. *Source:* MLHW of Japan (2017).

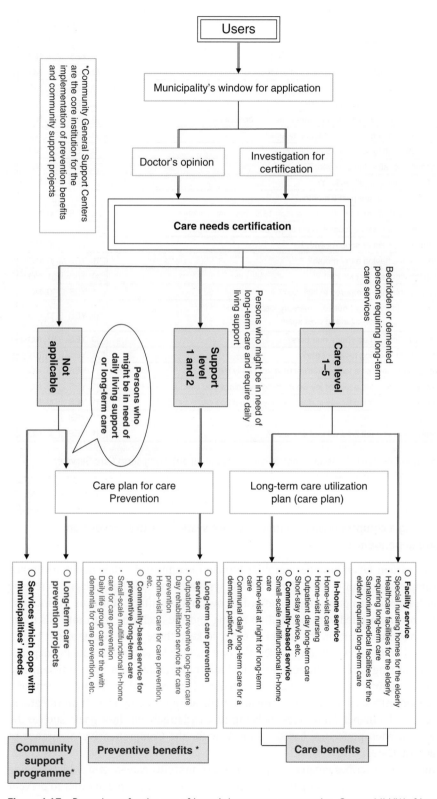

Figure 4.17 Procedures for the use of Japan's long-term care service. *Source:* MLHW of Japan (2017).

No.	Question	Answer	
1	Do you go out by bus or train by yourself?	☐0. YES	☐1. NO
2	Do you go shopping to buy daily necessities by yourself?	☐0. YES	☐1. NO
3	Do you manage your own deposits and savings at the bank?	☐0. YES	☐1. NO
4	Do you sometimes visit your friends?	☐0. YES	☐1. NO
5	Do you turn to your family or friends for advice?	☐0. YES	☐1. NO
6	Do you normally climb stairs without using handrail or wall for support?	☐0. YES	☐1. NO
7	Do you normally stand up from a chair without any aids?	☐0. YES	☐1. NO
8	Do you normally walk continuously for 15 minutes?	☐0. YES	☐1. NO
9	Have you experienced a fall in the past year?	☐1. YES	☐0. NO
10	Do you have a fear of falling while walking?	☐1. YES	☐0. NO
11	Have you lost 2 kg or more in the past 6 months?	☐1. YES	☐0. NO
12	Height: cm, Weight: kg, BMI: kg/m^2 If BMI is less than 18.5, this item is scored.	☐1. YES	☐0. NO
13	Do you have any difficulties eating tough foods compared to 6 months ago?	☐1. YES	☐0. NO
14	Have you choked on your tea or soup recently?	☐1. YES	☐0. NO
15	Do you often experience having a dry mouth?	☐1. YES	☐0. NO
16	Do you go out at least once a week?	☐0. YES	☐1. NO
17	Do you go out less frequently compared to last year?	☐1. YES	☐0. NO
18	Do your family or your friends point out your memory loss? e.g. "You ask the same question over and over again."	☐1. YES	☐0. NO
19	Do you make a call by looking up phone numbers?	☐0. YES	☐1. NO
20	Do you find yourself not knowing today's date?	☐1. YES	☐0. NO
21	In the last 2 weeks have you felt a lack of fulfillment in your daily life?	☐1. YES	☐0. NO
22	In the last 2 weeks have you felt a lack of joy when doing the things you used to enjoy?	☐1. YES	☐0. NO
23	In the last 2 weeks have you felt difficulty in doing what you could do easily before?	☐1. YES	☐0. NO
24	In the last 2 weeks have you felt helpless?	☐1. YES	☐0. NO
25	In the last 2 weeks have you felt tired without a reason?	☐1. YES	☐0. NO

Figure 4.18 The Kihon Checklist for assessment of care needs in Japan's Long-Term Care Service. *Source:* Arai H et al. 2015/John Wiley & Sons.

4.4.11 Establishing a comprehensive community care system for the prevention of long-term care dependence

Medical and dental care in Japan have been provided under the universal public health insurance system since its implementation in 1961. Japan's UHC system has enabled all citizens to receive medical and health services at a price they can afford for over half a century. However, the increase in social security costs associated with population ageing and the declining birth rate has made securing financial resources a major challenge. In order to keep these costs down, recent health reforms have focused on the prevention of NCDs, the prevention of frailty, and reducing dependence on long-term nursing care. Additional goals include transitioning to a more efficient and effective medical care delivery system based on the Medical Care Act and the establishment of a comprehensive community care system that provides medical and nursing care in an integrated manner at the local level. Financial resources are being allocated to achieve these goals, such as the creation of a fund for each prefecture based on the Law for the Comprehensive Assurance of Health and Long-term Care.

This section, therefore, describes Japan's comprehensive community care system, which is being established for the purpose of supporting the individual ADLs of older people in order to prevent

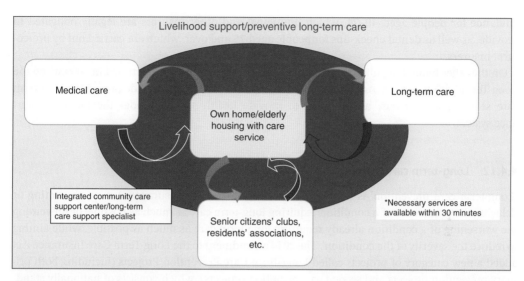

Figure 4.19 Integrated community care system of Japan. *Source:* Adapted from MHLW of Japan, Integrated community care system.

dependence on long-term care. In particular, the role of dental and oral health in this system will be discussed.

The MHLW described the comprehensive community care system as follows in its original proposal (Figure 4.19):

1) By 2025, when the baby-boomer generation is over 75 years old, a comprehensive community care system that provides housing, medical care, nursing care, prevention and lifestyle support in an integrated manner will be constructed so that people can continue living their own lives in their familiar communities to the end of their lives even if they become seriously in need of nursing care.

2) The number of elderly people with dementia is expected to increase in the future, so it is important to establish a comprehensive community care system to support the lives of elderly people with dementia in the community.

3) There are large regional differences in how population ageing is progressing. For example, in metropolitan areas the population is flat, but the number of people aged 75 and over is increasing rapidly. Meanwhile, in towns and villages, the population is decreasing, but the number of people aged 75 and over is increasing less rapidly. Regional comprehensive care systems need to be developed by municipalities and prefectures, which are the insurers, based on regional autonomy and independence, and in accordance with regional characteristics.

4) The community comprehensive care system is based on the concept of a 'daily life area' (similar to school districts for children), whereby necessary health services are accessible within approximately 30 minutes walking time from home.

In this system, the shift towards prevention in the public medical insurance system and long-term care insurance system is advanced. Preventive health services for individual patients are not covered under the public medical insurance system. Therefore, insurers are required to implement disease prevention activities under the Health Insurance Law and other laws. Preventive services provided in this way include specific health check-ups and specific health guidance for people aged 40–74, which municipal and other insurers are legally obligated to provide, as well as dental check-ups for people aged 75 and over, which are carried out by prefectural insurers.

On the other hand, the public long-term care insurance system, which started in 2000 when the Long-Term Care Insurance Act came into force, requires insurers to provide preventive long-term care services, just as they are required to provide health services under the medical insurance system.

4.4.12 Long-term care prevention

'Long-term care prevention' is defined in the Long-Term Care Insurance Act as 'preventing or delaying the occurrence of a condition requiring long-term care as much as possible or preventing the worsening of a condition already requiring long-term care as much as possible, while aiming to reduce the severity of the condition'. The 2014 amendment to the Long-Term Care Insurance Act added a new category of projects called Long-Term Care Prevention Projects (including both primary prevention projects and secondary prevention projects), which consists of nationally standardized preventive benefits (home-visit care and day-care services). Under this new category, population-based initiatives have been implemented, such as places for community residents to spend their time and socialize with each other.

Eligibility for this project is determined via a screening process based on the 'Kihon (Basic) Checklist', which consists of a 25-question interview (Figure 4.18), which assesses a person's physical (including oral) and mental condition, living environment and other elements that affect one's independence. In addition to determining eligibility, the responses to these questions are used to determine which services are provided to support each person's independence. In practice, Comprehensive Community Support Centres established in each region play a central role in ensuring that appropriate services suited to the situation of each person are provided in a comprehensive and efficient manner.

The Kihon (Basic) Checklist is a 25-item questionnaire developed to assess the life functions and degree of independence of older people and to predict the likelihood that they will require long-term care. Items 1–5 refer to activities of daily living, items 6–10 refer to motor functions, items 11 and 12 refer to nutrition, items 13–15 assess oral function, items 16 and 17 assess confinement, items 18–20 assess cognitive function and items 21–25 assess depression.

Programmes to prevent dependence on long-term care include:

1) **Motor function improvement programmes.** Physiotherapists, in collaboration with nursing care staff, implement activities such as aerobic exercise, stretching and exercises using simple equipment, which are designed to improve the functions of the locomotor organs and thereby improve life functions.

2) **Nutrition improvement programmes.** Dietitians, in collaboration with nursing care staff, prepare individual meal plans to improve the nutritional intake of older people. Based on these plans, individual nutritional consultations and group nutritional education sessions are provided to prevent health conditions associated with low nutritional intake.

3) **Oral function improvement programmes.** Dental hygienists, in collaboration with nursing and care staff, conduct eating and swallowing training, as well as tooth and tongue brushing training, in order to encourage improvement of oral functions (see more detailed information following this list).

4) **Combined programmes.** Integrated programmes, which combine the goals of improving musculoskeletal function, nutrition and oral function, are also implemented. These combined

programmes can be implemented depending on the needs and resources of each municipality, but they are highly recommended. For example, combining a nutrition improvement programme and an oral function improvement programme, or combining a motor function improvement programme and a nutrition improvement programme, have been shown to be highly effective.

5) **Other programmes.** Other programmes that are judged to be effective in preventing dependence on long-term care, such as programmes to prevent people from becoming shut-ins, prevent cognitive function decline, prevent depression and improve ADLs and IADLs (instrumental ADLs), can also be implemented at the municipal level.

Further details regarding the implementation of an 'oral function improvement programme' (point 2 in the preceding list) are as follows:

- Programme content – the objectives of the programme are education about the need to improve oral function, encouraging independence in cleaning the mouth, and improving eating and swallowing functions. The flow of the programme is determined according to the participants' condition. The implementation period is generally 3–6 months (the period and number of sessions should not impose an excessive burden on the users, but they should be sufficient to achieve results).
- Assessment – when providing oral function improvement services, the participants' condition should be ascertained via pre- and post-programme assessments. In addition, from a risk-assessment standpoint, the presence or absence of restrictions by doctors and dentists should be confirmed, and the presence or absence of pain in the oral cavity should also be checked. If there are complaints of pain during the assessment, or if the pain is noticeably above the standard level, dental professionals such as dentists and dental hygienists should be consulted as appropriate.
- Effectiveness of oral function improvement programmes – there have been reports of improvements in the oral environment and oral function after education about oral hygiene and oral function by professionals, and after training in oral hygiene procedures. Although there has been an increasing number of reports on the effectiveness of such oral function improvement programmes for older people, there have not yet been enough systematic reviews and meta-analyses published, so more evidence needs to be accumulated before conclusions can be drawn.

4.4.13 Proposal for improving home dental care provision

A study by Fukai (2007) assessed the dental care needs of the dependent elderly and proposed a short-term plan for the provision of home dental care in Japan.

It has been shown that Japanese people over age 75 with poor oral condition are reluctant to visit the dentist (MHLW of Japan 2020b) (Figure 4.20). The provision of home dental care is intended to help these people achieve oral health. However, only 18.2% of dental clinics currently provide home dental care, ranging from 11.0% in Okinawa Prefecture to 35.7% in Saga Prefecture. The percentage of dependent elderly who receive dental treatment at home is only 3.6%.

On the other hand, according to the 2005 national survey, there are 4 323 332 dependent elderly people out of a total of 25 672 005 people over age 65. The average number of dependent older people per dental clinic was 64.8, ranging from 35.9 in Tokyo to 133.6 in Shimane Prefecture.

Based on previous studies, the dental care needs of the dependent elderly can be classified into five categories: (1) to provide regular professional oral healthcare in order to prevent aspiration pneumonia for all dependent elderly; (2) to provide dental treatment for at least 50% of the dependent elderly; (3) to provide dysphagia rehabilitation to improve eating disorders for the

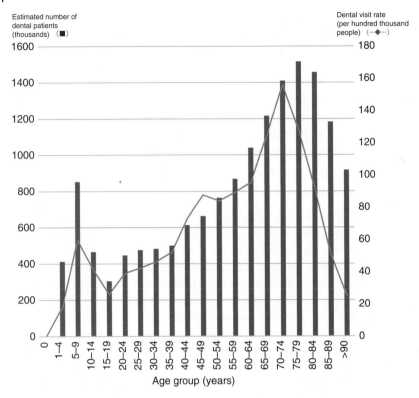

Figure 4.20 Pattern of dental visits by age group. *Source:* Adapted from MHLW of Japan (2020b).

dependent older adults; (4) to provide terminal dental care for patients at home; and (5) to provide dental care in hospitals.

To enhance the provision of these types of dental care, it is necessary to educate the public about the availability of home dental care, increase the number of dentists who specialize in home care, promote the involvement of dental clinics in community-based healthcare teams, and provide better incentives to dentists through the dental insurance system.

4.4.14 Provision of dental care under the Comprehensive Community Medical and Long-Term Care Fund

Dental care has been covered under Japan's NHI system since 1961. In 2003, a new publicly funded, long-term care insurance system was launched. This new system provides funding for municipalities to implement preventive oral-related services in order to prevent pneumonia as well as dependence on long-term care.

As the dental care provided under the NHI system was focused solely on outpatient care, people who are unable to visit a dental clinic had insufficient access to dental care. To address that need, home dental care as well as on-site dental care in hospitals and nursing homes is often touted as a new trend in dental care, but the reality on the ground is that only about 20% of dental clinics provide such services. This therefore remains a significant unmet need in Japan's dental care provision system.

In the next section, I start by discussing the current situation of home dental care in Japan. There is an effort under way to establish prefectural home dentistry centres from which care can be coordinated. This effort is being publicly funded, and it is separate from the NHI system. Then I discuss the progress that is being made toward providing dental care to the dependent elderly from a public health standpoint.

4.4.15 Dental examination and treatment in Japan

It is estimated that around 1.3 million Japanese people (1% of the population) visit a dentist each day. In the past year, about 60% of the population has visited a dental clinic.

The daily number of dental patients aged 65 and over was estimated at 310 000 (27.3% of all patients) in 2002, and this number doubled to 610 000 (45.4%) in a 2017 survey, meaning that nearly half of all dental patients are aged 65 and over (MHLW of Japan 2020b) (Figure 4.21). The dental expenditure for patients who are 65 and over is about 40% of the total dental expenditure, and this expenditure continues to increase as the number of elderly dental patients (and the proportion of the elderly who visit a dentist regularly) increases. The increasing proportion of elderly who visit dental clinics is a reflection of both increasing healthy longevity and an increasing number of teeth being maintained until an advanced age.

Although the provision of home dental care and dental care at non-dental healthcare facilities has been steadily increasing, there is a great deal of unmet need, particularly for the late-stage elderly (75 years old and over).

The baby-boomer generation will turn 75 years old around 2025, so the demand for medical, dental and nursing care among the late-stage elderly will increase significantly. For this reason, the national health policy in Japan is currently focused on developing a more efficient and high-quality medical care system as well as establishing regional comprehensive care systems. The most urgent

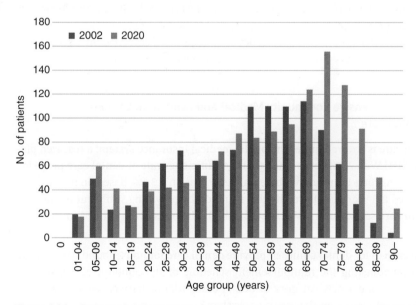

Figure 4.21 Estimated daily number of dental patients by age group, Japan. *Source:* Adapted from MHLW of Japan (2020b).

challenges in achieving those goals are: (1) flexible and efficient management of inpatient capacity; (2) promotion of home medical and nursing care; and (3) increasing the number medical and nursing care workers (by improving the working environment).

In the midst of these developments, the Comprehensive Community Medical and Long-Term Care Fund was established in each prefecture in 2014, utilizing the funds from the consumption tax increase. From that point on, each prefecture drew up its own plans and implemented its own projects to improve community-based healthcare services. The national government bears two-thirds of the financial burden, and prefectural governments bear the remaining third. The budget for this fund started at JPY90.4 billion for medical care in fiscal 2014, and additional expenditure was allotted for long-term nursing care the following year. By the 2021 budget, public expenditure through this fund had increased to JPY200.3 billion (JPY117.9 billion for medical care and JPY82.4 billion for long-term nursing care). Project categories supported by this fund are as follows:

1) Projects related to the improvement of medical facilities and equipment (including number and usage of beds) in accordance with achieve the Regional Medical Care Objectives (set by the national government).
2) Projects related to the provision of medical care in patients' homes or at nursing homes.
3) Projects related to the construction of local nursing homes and the improvement of existing facilities.
4) Projects related to the training and employment of community-based medical and nursing professionals.
5) Projects related to the training and employment of long-term care workers.
6) Projects related to reducing the working hours of hospital-employed physicians.

Under this programme, each prefecture draws up project proposals under the advice of prefectural healthcare associations and submits an application to the national government, which determines which projects to accept. Of the project categories listed above, categories 1 and 2 are most relevant to the provision of dental care. Under category 1, many prefectures have begun implementing projects that bring dental professionals into hospitals to provide dental care for in-patients in order reduce the duration of hospitalization. Under category 2, projects often employ dental professionals to provide dental care at patients' homes and at nursing homes.

4.4.16 Using the Comprehensive Community Medical and Long-Term Care Fund to promote home dental care

Although home dental care is covered under the public medical insurance system, a research project conducted by the MHLW in 2008 determined that the sufficiency rate of dental care provision for elderly people requiring long-term care with dental needs was only 3.6%. Based on this finding, the researchers proposed a 5-year plan to rectify this situation by providing sufficient dental care provision to long-term care service users (Fukai et al. 2007). The objectives outlined in that plan were as follows:

1) To increase the incentives for dental clinics to provide dental care for housebound patients and at nursing homes by adjusting the reimbursement schedule of the public health insurance system and also by creating a new category of dental clinic (domiciliary care-focused dental clinics) that can be registered under the insurance system.
2) To increase the provision of dental care in medical hospitals.

3) To establish an office in each prefecture staffed by personnel who can receive requests and arrange for the provision of dental care for housebound patients, in nursing homes and in hospitals. This also requires the establishment of a registry of participating dental clinics and professionals.

In order to develop a system to solve these problems, funding under the existing public medical insurance system was not sufficient, so additional prefectural-level and national-level government financial resources were necessary. With the establishment of the Comprehensive Community Medical and Long-Term Care Fund system in fiscal year 2014, a number of innovative initiatives utilizing this system have been implemented. For example, domiciliary dental care coordination offices have already been established in nearly all (44 prefectures) of Japan's 47 prefectures. These projects focus on providing consultation and referral services for prefectural residents and dental professionals, maintenance and provision of domiciliary care equipment, and recruiting dental hygienists (MHLW of Japan 2022d) (Figure 4.22). These home dental care coordination offices will become the foundation for meeting the needs for dental care and multidisciplinary collaboration in the context of regional comprehensive care systems by 2025, and some prefectures are already beginning to establish such offices in multiple locations or municipalities within the prefecture.

The lesson to be learned from Japan's experience in this area is that in order to improve the provision of dental care, including providing adequate domiciliary dental care, it was necessary to position dental care not only as the responsibility of individual dental institutions compensated by the public insurance system, but also as an integral and indispensable part of a comprehensive public health infrastructure. While it is impossible to require dental clinics and professionals to provide home dental care, it is possible to reduce the barriers and increase the incentives for them to do so.

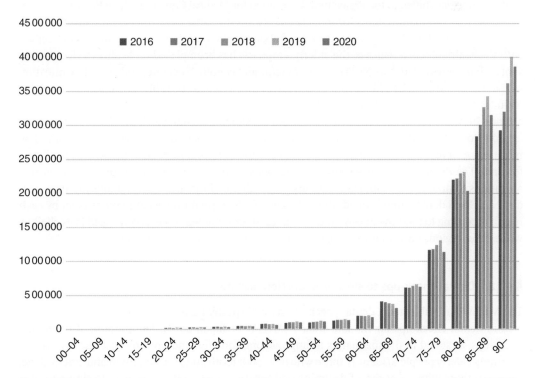

Figure 4.22 Changes in the number of home dental care provision fee calculations, Japan. *Source:* MHLW of Japan (2022d).

4.4.17 Health services and dental examinations for the late stage older adults (75 years and older)

Extending HLE is a major goal of Japan's health policy. The primary target is the prevention of NCDs such as heart disease, cancer and diabetes, as well as prevention of frailty and long-term care dependence (see Figure 4.10). Disease prevention in Japan is based on the Maternal and Child Health Act, the School Health and Safety Act, the Health Promotion Act, the Medical Insurance Act, the Act on Securing Medical Care for the Elderly, and the Long-Term Care Insurance Act.

The Medical Insurance Act and the Act on Securing Medical Care for the Elderly require insurers not only to provide benefits for disease treatment, but also to provide public health services such as dental check-ups and health guidance. In addition, the Long-Term Care Insurance Act requires municipalities to become insurers and provide public health services designed to prevent long-term care dependence. In this section, I discuss the role of dental check-ups conducted by an insurer called the Prefectural Association for Medical Care for the Late Elderly (operating in all 47 prefectures) in promoting dental health. I also introduce the system of specific health check-ups and specific health guidance (40–74 years old) that has been implemented based on the Act on Securing Medical Care for the Elderly.

The Prefectural Association for Medical Care of the Late Elderly must strive to conduct health services such as health education, health consultations and health check-ups that are deemed necessary for the retention and promotion of the health of insured persons. These services are funded by the insurer (two-thirds) and federal government subsidies (one-third). Municipalities were required to conduct health check-ups for the late stage older adults (75 years and older) under the former Geriatric Health Law, but since the establishment of the medical care system for the late elderly in 2008, this responsibility has shifted to the Prefectural Association for Medical Care of the Late Elderly.

The health examination items for the late elderly are the same as for the specific health check-ups for ages 40–74, excluding measurement of abdominal circumference. In addition, in keeping with the health characteristics of the elderly, emphasis has been placed on health services to prevent serious illnesses such as NCDs, prevent motor and cognitive decline, and avoid low nutrition so that the elderly can live independent daily lives for as long as possible. The questionnaire also includes items related to oral function (MHLW of Japan 2019).

Since 2014, the federal government also began subsidizing dental check-ups for the late elderly in order to prevent ADLs from declining due to poor oral function, pneumonia, frailty and low nutrition. As a result, dental check-ups for the late elderly have now been implemented in all prefectures. The dental check-up system is the responsibility of the regional insurers, who entrust operations to prefectural dental associations. The individual medical examinations are then conducted at local dental clinics. In addition, the age of eligibility for the examinations is set by each region according to their own needs and resources, so in some regions everyone aged 75 is eligible, while other regions only offer the check-ups at certain ages, such as 75 and 80.

4.4.18 Dental check-ups to slow oral function decline

The MHLW has published a dental check-up manual specifying the examination items to be covered in dental check-ups for the late elderly (MHLW of Japan 2018). The purpose of the dental check-ups, as stated in the manual, is to improve oral function and prevent systemic diseases by screening elderly people to identify those who have poor tooth and gum condition and oral hygiene, as well as those who are at risk of declining oral function, in order to refer them to clinics for further examinations and treatment.

The recommended items to be included in these dental check-ups are (1) assessment of oral function ('masticatory function', 'tongue/lip function', 'swallowing function') via one of a number of prescribed assessment methods (each region can choose the method that best fits their needs and resources), and (2) medical interviews regarding medication, living situation, as well as possible indicators of low nutrition and aspiration pneumonia, such as weight loss and fever. The responses to these interviews are used by insurers to identify those at high risk for frailty, who can then be provided with appropriate follow-up care such as health guidance.

People who are assessed as having poor oral function or being at high risk for declining oral function are referred to dental clinics for further and/or more detailed dental examinations as well as health guidance. At that point, if there is a diagnosis requiring dental treatment, the treatment is covered under the public health insurance system.

In order to facilitate public insurance coverage of measures to slow oral function decline oral function, its pathophysiology was described by the Japanese Dental Science Association in 2018. It was defined as a state in which the function of the oral cavity is reduced, whether due to ageing or specific diseases and disorders (e.g. caries, periodontology, tooth loss, denture incompatibility). If left untreated, declining oral function leads to masticatory dysfunction and dysphagia, thereby damaging systemic health. The relationship between oral function and systemic health is bidirectional: low nutrition, disuse syndrome, side-effects of drugs and complex disease state are risk factors for declining oral function.

Therefore, it is necessary to manage oral function in a way that takes into account the living environment and general condition of individual elderly people. Oral function decline is diagnosed if a patient presents with three of the following seven sub-symptoms: poor oral hygiene, dryness of the oral cavity, reduced bite force, reduced lip movement, reduced tongue pressure, decreased masticatory function and reduced swallowing function. A management plan is determined after diagnosis, and reassessment is conducted via examination approximately every 6 months.

Frailty progresses much more rapidly in late elderly people compared with the earlier stage of old age. In addition, since comorbidities such as multiple chronic diseases and geriatric syndrome are also likely to be present, comprehensive disease management is required. In the dental field, which has focused mainly on outpatient care, the treatment rate has tended to decrease after the age of 75; however, it also increases with an increasing number of remaining teeth. In addition, home dental care is also being advanced as part of current national health policy.

In line with Japanese national policy goals, there is growing awareness that dental care for the elderly is an essential element of preventive medical care that helps delay the decline in the living functions of the elderly. In addition, as most dental and oral health professionals are situated in local dental clinics, it is predicted that health policies that utilize this manpower to its fullest potential will help to reduce health disparities while at the same time preventing and reducing oral diseases and tooth loss from early childhood and throughout the life course.

4.4.19 The role of dental care and oral health in dementia policies and measures in Japan

Dementia is an unavoidable health issue in ageing societies. In Japan, it is estimated that there will be approximately 7 million people with dementia (accounting for 1 in 5 of the elderly population) by 2025. In 2012, the number was 4.62 million (1 in 7 of the elderly population). This section describes dementia policies and measures in Japan and the role of dental and oral health therein.

4.4.19.1 Comprehensive plan to promote dementia measures (New Orange Plan)

The MHLW formulated and promoted its 'Five-Year Plan for Promoting Dementia Measures (Orange Plan)', which was intended to be in effect during the period 2013–2017. However, dementia is a global issue, not just a national issue, and in 2013 the G8 Dementia Summit was held in the UK to begin developing a global strategy. A follow-up event was then held in Tokyo in November 2014, and I participated in that event as a representative from the field of dental and oral health. In the aftermath of that event, a new comprehensive strategy for promoting dementia measures (New Orange Plan) was announced by the government in January 2015 (MHLW of Japan 2015).

The New Orange Plan is in effect until 2025, when baby boomers will be elderly. The objective of this plan is to realize a society where people living with dementia are treated with respect and are able to continue living well and in the manner they are used to, and, to the extent possible, in the environment with which they are most familiar and comfortable. This new plan consists of the following seven core aims:

1) To promote heightened awareness of dementia through the dissemination of information.
2) To provide medical treatment and long-term care that is timely and appropriate to the patient's dementia status.
3) To strengthen policies and provisions for early-onset dementia.
4) To support those who provide long-term care to people living with dementia.
5) To promote the realization of an elderly-friendly and dementia-friendly society.
6) To promote research on the prevention, diagnosis and treatment of dementia as well as rehabilitation and long-term care models, and to promote dissemination of the evidence and findings that arise from such research.
7) To respect the perspective of people living with dementia and their families.

In the Orange Plan of 2013, dentists were given an important role in early detection and early response to dementia. In the New Orange Plan, revised in 2015, the necessity of improving the ability of dentists to play this role was clarified, and, as part of a research project conducted by the MHLW in 2015, a training text was created for dentists nationwide. Since 2016, such training programmes have been conducted in each prefecture in line with this programme.

In addition to this, the positioning of dental clinics in dementia care paths is being promoted in each prefecture. In 2019, the Guidelines for Dental Care for Dementia Patients were issued as part of the national budget, based on scientific evidence showing the association between dementia and oral health. In this way, efforts to standardize the dementia response in dental care are advancing in the context of national dementia policy.

4.4.19.2 The role of dental and oral health in dementia prevention

At all life stages, the purpose of dental care is to reduce symptoms associated with dental disease and tooth loss, maintain and restore oral function, and prevent or delay the onset and progression of dental diseases, both for healthy people and for those with diseases and disabilities. All people have a fundamental human right to receive support for the retention of oral function, including eating, until the final stages of life.

Family dentists in community settings see the same patients regularly over long periods of time, so one of our important responsibilities as healthcare providers is to notice the signs of dementia onset at an early stage. There is still some anxiety among dental professionals regarding the provision of care for patients living with dementia, and many such professionals still have an inadequate understanding of the pathophysiology of dementia. There is also still a lack of guidelines for dental treatment of patients with dementia. Regardless of this situation, however, as healthcare professionals, dentists and dental hygienists do have an important role to play in national dementia measures, and as part of that role we need to deepen our understanding of dementia.

At this point I would also like to clarify the role of dental care and oral health in preventing and delaying the onset of dementia. Long-term follow-up studies have reported that the retention of natural teeth, bite force and masticatory functions contribute to preventing the onset of dementia. In addition, epidemiological studies such as the Hisayama-cho Study (Ozawa et al. 2013; Ninomiya 2018) have shown the effect of a good diet on the prevention of dementia through analysis of types of food ingested. As research reports showing the relationship between tooth loss and food intake have accumulated, the role of dental care and oral health in preventing dementia has become clearer, particularly in the context of the life course approach.

4.4.20 The Metabolic Syndrome Screening System and oral health

Non-communicable diseases such as cancer, heart disease, cerebrovascular disease, diabetes mellitus and hypertension account for approximately 60% of deaths and 30% of medical expenses in Japan. Therefore, nationally coordinated NCD prevention measures have great potential to extend HLE.

At the same time, dental care is provided to more than 1.3 million people (1% of the population) every day, and among adults visiting the dentist for the first time, 20.7% have hypertension, 5.8% have diabetes, 3.5% have heart disease, and 1.8% have cancer (Fukai et al. 2019b). Moreover, dental patients tend to visit a dental clinic regularly over a long period of time, so in many cases they will have been visiting a dental clinic both before and after the incidence of the NCD.

Due to the relationship between oral health and general health, and the fact that oral health contributes to extended HLE, a policy framework that links public NCD prevention measures with dental care is needed. With this in mind, Japan has enacted a system whereby the national health insurers are legally required to implement specific health check-ups and health guidance aimed at the prevention of metabolic syndrome for all insured persons between the ages of 40 and 74. Under this system there are a total of 53 million insured persons insured by 3365 insurers, so positioning dental clinics in this system would have a huge effect on NCD prevention.

4.4.21 Public health policy for NCD prevention

Japan's first national health promotion campaign was enacted in 1978, and the first comprehensive set of concrete health promotion goals related to NCDs, Health Japan 21, was enacted in 2000. That national project continues today, now in its second stage, and prevention of NCDs is still one of the most important goals for extending HLE and reducing health disparities; dental and oral health are positioned as essential elements of that effort.

In addition, a national system of specific health check-ups and health guidance for the prevention of metabolic syndrome was implemented in April 2008 (MHLW of Japan 2018b). Unhealthy lifestyle behaviour related to exercise, diet, smoking, and so on are known to contribute to obesity, lipid abnormality, high blood sugar and high blood pressure, which in turn are associated with the onset and progression of ischaemic heart disease, cerebrovascular disease, diabetes mellitus, and the like. Therefore, from a public health standpoint, the most effective preventive measures involve implementing a screening system to identify people with high risk at an early stage, before the disease becomes severe, and offering those people individual health education and consultation by healthcare professionals.

An important characteristic of this system is that it includes a systematic outcome assessment phase which involves analysing data from over 25 million anonymized medical examinations. These data are automatically registered in the National Database run by the MHLW and used to assess both the implementation and results of the check-up and guidance system.

Since the introduction of this system, health education materials designed to prevent metabolic syndrome (diabetes, obesity and heart disease prevention) have been developed and distributed to dentists and dental hygienists, along with a training requirement, so that they can provide specific health guidance that goes beyond the traditional scope of dental and oral health.

The national system of specific health check-ups and health guidance is reviewed and updated once every 5 years. In the most recent update (for 2018–2023), question items regarding subjective chewing function were added because decline in chewing function is indicative of dental disease and tooth loss. Another revision was that dentists are no longer required to undergo training in order to provide dietary improvement guidance.

As a result, the current role of dental institutions in the system of specific health check-ups and health guidance is as follows:

1) Those who are identified as having potential dental problems based on the questionnaire results are encouraged to visit a dental clinic for examination. Dental health guidance is then provided to patients who visit clinics.
2) Those who are identified as having chewing function decline are encouraged to visit a dental clinic to receive chewing improvement guidance. Dental clinics then receive compensation from the national insurers for providing such guidance.
3) Dental clinics can also offer specific health guidance for those who have been flagged (via the screening system) for potential metabolic syndrome if they have entered into a contract with the national insurers. Such guidance would focus on metabolic syndrome risk reduction and can be provided by dentists or dental hygienists; an outcome assessment must be performed by a nutritionist, physician or nurse.

The role in point 3 in the preceding list represents the clearest and strongest contribution by dental clinics to metabolic syndrome prevention, but it is also the most difficult for most clinics to achieve, particularly because they must hire a nutritionist, at least part time. Some clinics, however, such as the author's, have already begun taking on this role (Fukai 2019). Beginning in 2019, the Saitama Prefectural Dental Association signed an agreement with national insurers to enable registered dental clinics in the prefecture to offer this type of health guidance.

In order to achieve a healthy ageing society, the most effective target for public health measures is NCD prevention and the prevention of frailty and long-term care dependence. As we have seen in Chapter 3, a rich body of accumulated evidence indicates a strong association between oral health and both NCDs and frailty, including many common risk factors. For this reason, there is a great deal of overlap between the health education content for oral disease prevention and NCD/frailty prevention. This means that a multi-sectoral, common risk factor approach in which both dental professionals and medical professionals provide standardized NCD and frailty prevention education is the most effective (and cost-effective) system. Another way of looking at it is that dental clinics should be put to work as social capital, contributing to disease prevention and thereby healthy longevity. Breaking down the walls between the health professions in this way would improve access and reduce some of the inequities inherent in the current healthcare system, and doing so systematically at the national level would be the most efficient way of achieving this.

4.4.22 Japan's 8020 Campaign

The 8020 Campaign for oral health promotion, whose goal is to encourage people to keep 20 of their own teeth until the age of 80, is a national oral health campaign that has been carried out for the past three decades by the Japanese government and the Japan Dental Association (JDA).

In 1989, Japan's Ministry of Health and Welfare (MHW) launched the 8020 Campaign to encourage people to keep 20 or more of their natural teeth until the age of 80. At the time, only 7% of 80-year-olds had 20 or more teeth. The campaign turned out to be much more successful than expected, with the percentage of those achieving 80–20 status increasing steadily through 2016, when over half of 80-year-olds had achieved it.

As Japan's population began rapidly ageing in the 1970s and 1980s, this campaign was implemented in order to provide comprehensive and high-quality dental healthcare for older adults and the elderly, for whom such services had not previously been sufficiently provided. In tandem with other health policies enacted at the time, it was thought that this campaign would establish an easy-to-understand goal towards which to strive, and that such a goal would in turn lead to improved oral health in elderly people. It was hoped that establishing this goal would have a positive washback effect that would motivate both individuals and oral health professionals to work together to establish preventive measures to maintain oral health at all stages of life.

The campaign adopted a broad-based life course approach to preventing tooth loss by engaging multiple sectors and carrying out initiatives that targeted all generations (MHLW of Japan 2012). The MHLW provided subsidies to local governments and dental associations to carry out various oral health initiatives, which included providing check-ups (including oral health guidance) for expecting mothers and young children between 1.5 and 3 years old, as well as for individuals over the ages of 40, 50, 60 and 80 years (MHLW of Japan 2020). Table 4.1 provides a timeline of the 8020 Campaign from 1989 to 1999. The Ministry of Education, Culture, Sports, Science and

Table 4.1 History of the 8020 Campaign (1989–1999).

1989	The MHW's 'Group to Consider Adult Dental Health Measures' published its interim report, in which the 8020 Campaign was proposed.
1991	Promotion of the 8020 Campaign was established as one of the priority goals for Dental Health Week.
1991	The MHW started a project to promote the 8020 Campaign as one of its new budget subsidy projects.
1992	A WHO panel of experts on recent progress in oral health included a description of the 8020 Campaign in its report.
1993	The JDA set up a meeting to consider the promotion of the 8020 Campaign.
1994	The JDA's meeting to consider the promotion of the 8020 Campaign published its report.
1995	Periodontal disease examination was added to the list of general health examination items.
1996	The JDA's Public Health Committee drew up a report on the promotion of the 8020 Campaign.
1997	Special projects to promote the 8020 Campaign were launched by municipal governments and Tokyo's 23 ward governments.
1998	The JDA established a committee to consider establishing an 8020 Promotion Foundation.
1999	The JDA's committee to consider establishing an 8020 Promotion Foundation (tentative name) put together a report.

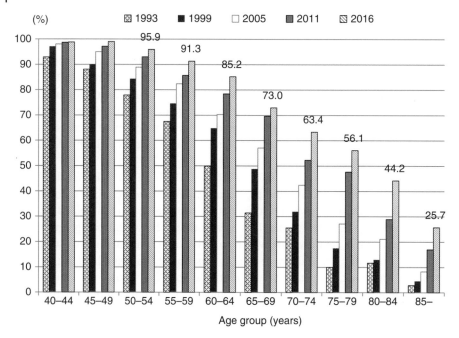

Figure 4.23 Percentage of individuals with over 20 teeth remaining. *Source:* Data from MHLW of Japan (2016).

Technology also provided school-based initiatives such as annual check-ups for students between 6 and 18 years old by school dentists and school-based fluoride mouth-rinsing programmes for children and adolescents aged 4–14 years.

In 2000, the 8020 Promotion Foundation was established to conduct research related to the campaign and raise awareness. The MHLW carried out a national survey of dental diseases in 2016 and found that 51% of 80-year-olds in Japan had more than 20 teeth, meaning that the campaign had reached its goal six years before the target year of 2022 (Figure 4.23). The prevalence of tooth decay among children had also decreased as a result of the campaign activities, which specifically addressed oral health in children (MHLW of Japan 2016). Finally, the research conducted by the 8020 Promotion Foundation provided the impetus for the 'Act on the Promotion of Dental and Oral Health' in 2011, which further reinforced the importance of oral health promotion.

4.4.22.1 History of the 8020 Campaign

Tables 4.1 and 4.2 provide a full timeline of the 8020 Campaign. The campaign was first proposed by the MHW as the central initiative of the 1991 Dental Health Week. The campaign at that time consisted primarily of providing financial support for prefectural governments' oral health promotion activities.

In 1993, JDA started discussing the successes and future prospects of the 8020 Campaign, gradually developing a consensus around continuing and expanding its scope. These discussions led to the first official report on the campaign being issued in 1994, and in 2000 the 8020 Promotion Foundation was established. This foundation engaged in promotional activities, educational

Table 4.2 History of the 8020 Campaign (2000–).

2000	The Health Japan 21 project (first phase) was launched.
	Special projects to promote the 8020 Campaign were launched by prefectural governments with new MHW subsidies.
	The 8020 Promotion Foundation was established.
2002	The Health Promotion Act was enacted.
2004	People aged 60 and 70 were added to the list of those who should undergo examinations for periodontal disease as part of health promotion projects for the elderly.
2007	Periodontal disease examinations were included in the examination items stipulated in the Health Promotion Act.
2008	The late elderly healthcare system, which encouraged dental clinics to provide home dental care, was implemented.
	An official ceremony and symposiums were held to commemorate the 20th anniversary of the 8020 Campaign.
2011	The Act Concerning the Promotion of Dental and Oral Health was enacted.
2012	'Basic Matters Related to the Promotion of Dental and Oral Health' was published.
	The national health promotion policy, Health Japan 21 (second phase), was launched.
2013	The MHLW started its oral health promotion projects.
2014	The MHLW launched a project to subsidize insurers when providing dental examinations for people aged 75 or older.
2019	An official ceremony and symposiums to commemorate the 30th anniversary of the 8020 Campaign were held.

projects and research subsidization designed to expand the campaign to local communities in every region of Japan.

Originally, when the campaign was launched by the JDA and the dental section of the MHW, emphasis was placed on nationwide promotion of the campaign itself, gathering and disseminating information about the campaign's activities and successes at the local level, and assessing the campaign's effectiveness. The campaign has been widely recognized as one of the most successful modern public health initiatives in Japan and it now holds a solid position in national health policy.

Based on the success of this campaign, the scope of dental and oral health research is now expanding beyond the examination of individual dental diseases to include research on the contribution of oral health to the prevention of NCDs and other health issues (such as frailty) related to healthy longevity. Against this backdrop, in 2013 the 8020 Promotion Foundation published recommendations highlighting the need for policies that focus on providing heightened funding for research projects that integrate oral health and general healthcare, in addition to those that focus solely on dental care provision.

Another milestone in the timeline, which served to strengthen and expand the 8020 Campaign, was the Act Concerning the Promotion of Dental and Oral Health, established in 2011. The road to realizing this law was a long one. Since the 1950s there had been several waves of growing interest in enacting it, and dental and healthcare professionals had long hoped for such legislation. In the following year, an action plan called, 'Basic Matters Related to the Promotion of Dental and Oral Health' was initiated. At the same time, a national health promotion policy called Health Japan 21

Table 4.3　Health Japan 21 (second phase), 2013–2023.

Indicators	Baseline data	Interim evaluation (2017)	Target
① **Maintenance and improvement of oral function (increase in percentage of individuals in their 60s with good mastication)**	73.4% (2009)	72.6% (2016)	80% (2022)
② **Prevention of tooth loss**			
(a) Increase in percentage of 80-year-old individuals with over 20 teeth remaining	25.0% (2005)	51.2% (2016)	50%⇒60% (2022)
(b) Increase in percentage of 60-year-old individuals with over 24 teeth remaining	60.2% (2005)	74.4% (2016)	70%⇒80% (2022)
(c) Increase in percentage of 40-year-old individuals with all teeth remaining	54.1% (2005)	73.4% (2016)	75% (2022)
③ **Decrease in percentage of individuals with periodontal disease**			
(a) Decrease in percentage of individuals in 20s with gingivitis	31.7% (2009)	27.1% (2014)	25% (2022)
(b) Decrease in percentage of individuals in 40s with progressive periodontitis	37.3% (2005)	44.7% (2016)	25% (2022)
(c) Decrease in percentage of individuals in 60s with progressive periodontitis	54.7% (2005)	59.4% (2016)	45% (2022)
④ **Increase in number of children without dental caries**			
(a) Increase in number of prefectures where over 80% of 3-year-old children have no dental caries	6 prefectures (2009)	26 prefectures (2015)	23 prefectures⇒47 (2022)
(b) Increase in number of prefectures where 12-year-old children have less than 1 DMFT	7 prefectures (2011)	28 prefectures (2016)	28 prefectures⇒47 (2022)
⑤ **Increase in percentage of individuals who participated in dental check-up during the past year**	34.1% (2009)	52.9% (2016)	65% (2022)

DMFT: sum of the number of decayed, missing due to caries, and filled teeth in the permanent teeth.
Source: Ministry of Health, Labour and Welfare of Japan.

(second phase) was launched, establishing the goal of increasing the percentage of people with 20 teeth at the age of 80 to 50% by 2023 (Table 4.3). These initiatives resulted in the formulation of new dental health and dental care programmes as well as the setting of concrete goals expressed in terms of oral functions.

The MHLW then proceeded to subsidize new projects related to cooperation between medicine and dentistry. Oral health promotion projects aimed at developing oral health centres in each prefecture and in major cities were also subsidized.

4.4.22.2 Expanding the role of the 8020 Campaign

When the campaign was initiated, the primary goal was to improve the eating behaviour and QOL of elderly people. However, the evidence that has accumulated since that time now clearly shows a link between number of teeth and general health. As a result, the goal of 20 teeth by 80 years of age has been officially recognized as a national health goal for achieving healthy longevity in Japan.

Although more than 50% of 80-year-olds have already achieved the 8020 goal, it is necessary to further improve dental care and oral health in order to realize a society that is truly characterized by healthy longevity. The previous goal of increasing the number of remaining teeth was simple and worked extremely well, but it is now necessary to establish new assessment indicators and new goals from the perspective of enhancing oral function as well as maintaining daily living functions. In order to prevent tooth loss, the current community-based campaign needs to be accompanied by regular dental care and treatment, so the 8020 Campaign also needs to be promoted in dental clinics in the years to come. Moreover, the Act Concerning the Promotion of Dental and Oral Health stipulates that necessary measures should be taken to ensure access to dental care for people with disabilities and others who have difficulty accessing it. It is imperative that dental organizations, including the 8020 Promotion Foundation, further develop the projects they have implemented up to now and recommend new policies for improving dental and oral health. We need to further promote the 8020 Campaign, not only in the context of community health programmes but also in the context of regular dental care. We also need to position the campaign as part of the effort to promote general health in cooperation with other health professionals.

The MHLW stated in the 'Basic Matters Related to the Promotion of Dental and Oral Health' of July 2012 that the goal of the 8020 Campaign was not only to improve oral health but also to improve general health. It is therefore essential to consider ways to offer the best mix of oral health and general health services and dental care provision while taking into consideration the relationship between the campaign and medical services.

From the experience of this Japanese campaign, other countries can gain insights on how to engage in their own process of developing dental health policy.

4.4.22.3 Effects of the 8020 Campaign on public health

There have been many studies investigating the association between oral health and general health, and evidence on this relationship continues to accumulate (see Chapter 3).

Regarding the relationship between oral health and diabetes, for example, many intervention studies have suggested that periodontal disease increases blood sugar levels; therefore, treatment of periodontitis results in improved blood glucose control. A study conducted by Yoneyama et al. (1999) on the institutionalized older adults indicated that intensive oral care reduced the number of the participants who developed fever or pneumonia or died from pneumonia. They also found that oral care was effective in preventing aspiration pneumonia.

Furthermore, the results of a 15-year cohort study carried out on Miyakojima Island, Okinawa Prefecture showed that elderly people who retained a higher number of functional teeth had a higher survival rate (Fukai et al. 2007). It also showed that people with fewer functional teeth were more likely to complain about physical conditions such as pain in their lower back, shoulders and upper and lower limbs. Other studies have found that older people undergoing dental care are less likely to suffer from declining physical functions which would reduce their ADLs and lead them to depend on nursing care (Fukai et al. 2009).

In August 2013, Japan's MHLW published its vision to achieve a 'society where the healthy life of people is extended,' along with a variety of health care initiatives such as prophylaxis funding. The ministry aims to achieve these goals by providing oral care in combination with preventive care for aspiration pneumonia in the elderly and by preventing the progression of diabetes through health examinations and health guidance, including treatment of periodontal diseases. There is a need for further research ascertaining the effects of the 8020 Campaign on general health.

4.5 Conclusion

Any national UHC system needs to take into account the financial burden and to make effective and efficient use of human resources in the health sector. Cross-sectoral collaboration is therefore required, and it is effective to include oral health programmes in overall health policy, rather than having an isolated policy that is specific to dental and oral health. As health systems differ in each country, it is advisable to build on and make use of the strengths of each system and for countries to share and learn from each other's UHC initiatives. Access to essential oral health services throughout life is a fundamental human right that should be ensured in every region and in every country.

The realization of a 'society of longevity' is a result of human advancement and therefore something to be celebrated. On the other hand, the decline of vital functions and health with age is something we cannot avoid biologically. To address this seemingly paradoxical issue, we urgently need to develop a social structure and healthcare system that will allow elderly individuals to lead their lives with purpose and dignity. To this end, specific measures can and must be taken to reduce health inequalities among generations and regions, thereby extending HLE in each and every individual.

Since the implementation of a universal health insurance system in 1961, the health status of the people of Japan has improved considerably and the country has achieved a level of longevity greater than anywhere else in the world. As the nation standing at the forefront of the global society of longevity, Japan has a responsibility to report its experiences to the world, particularly concerning its healthcare policies and campaigns as well as our ongoing attempts to reform the system.

As the evidence and analyses presented in this publication confirm, basic dental and oral functionality is associated with self-expression and socialization – which are fundamental human rights – through diet and communication. In the long run, dental and oral health is also associated with vital prognosis in humans. In fact, an accumulation of evidence suggests that dental care and oral health can and do contribute to the realization of healthy longevity.

Against this backdrop, and based on the analyses in this book, I make the following recommendations regarding healthy longevity, dental care and oral health:

1) Health and medical care systems should be developed in such a way that even in old age, anyone can receive the dental care and oral health services they need, no matter where they live.
2) Dental health care personnel should make continuous efforts to communicate the current evidence regarding dental care, oral health and healthy longevity to citizens and health policymakers.

3) The development of health and medical technology should be promoted, in addition to training human resources that provide evidence-based health and medical services.

4) Dental healthcare personnel and relevant organizations should work together to enact measures that target the risk factors which are common to both oral diseases and NCDs, and they should also work to develop health systems based on a continuous life-course approach covering the period from adulthood to old age.

5) High-quality research should be conducted to accumulate evidence which further clarifies the causal relationship linking dental and oral health to healthy longevity.

6) Evidence-based health policies which reflect the association between dental and oral health and the extension of HLE should be implemented, and studies verifying the effectiveness of these policies should be undertaken.

References

Fukai, K., Furuta, M., Shimazaki, Y. et al. (2017). The oral health and general health of Japanese community residents: The 8020 Promotion Foundation Study on the Health Promotion Effects of Dental Care. *Journal of the Japanese Association for Dental Science*, 36, 62–73.

Aida, J., Fukai, K., & Watt, R. (2020). Global neglect of dental coverage in universal health coverage systems and Japan's broad coverage. *Int D J Int Dent J*, 71(6), 454–457.

Aida, J., Takeuchi, K., Furuta, M. et al. (2022). Burden of oral diseases and access to oral care in an ageing society. *Int Dent J*, 72(4S), S5–S11.

Arai, H., Satake, S. (2015). English translation of the Kihon Checklist. *Geriatric Gerontol Int*, 15(4), 518–519.

Chávez, E.M., Kossioni, A., & Fukai, K. (2022). Policies supporting oral health in ageing populations are needed worldwide. *Int Dent J*, 72(4S), S27–S38. https://www.ncbi.nlm.nih.gov/pmc/articles/PMC9437798/pdf/main.pdf (accessed 13 May 2024).

FDI. (2023). *Access to Oral Health through Primary Health Care*. White paper. Geneva: FDI. https://www.fdiworlddental.org/sites/default/files/2023–05/FDI%20Access%20to%20Oral%20Health%20Care%20White%20Paper.pdf (accessed 13 May 2024).

Fukai, K. (2007). Assessing the dental care needs of the dependent elderly and a short-term plan of the provision of home dental care in Japan. *Health Sci Health Care*, 7, 88–107.

Fukai, K. (2019). Oral health for healthy aging society -evidence and health policy. *JJHEP*, 27(4), 360–368.

Fukai, K., Furuta, M., Aida, J. et al. (2019b). Association between oral health and general health of Japanese dental patients: The 8020 Promotion Foundation Study on the Health Promotion Effects of Dental Care: A 3-year cohort study. *Journal of the Japanese Association for Dental Science*, 38, 84–93.

Fukai, K., Takiguchi, T., Ando, Y. et al. (2007). Functional tooth number and 15-year mortality in a cohort of community-residing older people. *Geriatr Gerontol Int*, 7, 341–347.

Fukai, K., Takiguchi, T., Ando, Y. et al. (2009). Associations between functional tooth number and physical complaints of community residing adults in a 15-year cohort study. *Geriatr Gerontol Int*, 9, 366–371.

Fukai, K. Furuta, M., Shimazaki, Y. et al. (2014). The oral and general health of Japanese community resident: The 8020 Promotion Foundation Study on the health promotion effects of dental care. *J Jap Assoc Dental Sci*, 36, 62–73.

Fukai, K., Ogawa, H., & Hescot, P. (2017). Oral health for healthy longevity in an ageing society: Maintaining momentum and moving forward. *Int Dent J*, 67(Suppl 2), 3–6.

Global Burden of Disease Study (GBD) 2019 Universal Health Coverage Collaborators. (2020). Measuring universal health coverage based on an index of effective coverage of health services in 204 countries and territories, 1990–2019: a systematic analysis for the Global Burden of Disease Study 2019. *Lancet*, 396(10258), 1250–1284.

Harris, RV. (2013). Operationalisation of the construct of access to dental care: a position paper and proposed conceptual definitions. *Community Dent Health.* 30(2), 94–101.

Hart, J.T. (1971). The inverse care law. *Lancet*, 297(7696), 405–412.

Ikegami N. (2014). *Universal Health Coverage for Inclusive and Sustainable Development Lessons from Japan*. World Bank. https://elibrary.worldbank.org/doi/book/10.1596/978–1–4648–0408–3?chapterTab=true (accessed 13 May 2024).

Ikegami, N., Yoo, B.K., Hashimoto, H. et al. (2011). Japanese universal health coverage: evolution, achievements, and challenges. *Lancet*, 17, 378(9796), 1106–1115.

Kieny, M.P., Bekedam, H., Dovlo, D. et al. (2017). Strengthening health systems for universal health coverage and sustainable development. *Bull World Health Organ*, 95(8), 608.

Maeda, A. et al. (2014). Universal Health Coverage for Inclusive and Sustainable Development A Synthesis of 11 Country Case Studies Washington, DC, The World Bank https://documents1.worldbank.org/curated/en/575211468278746561/pdf/888620PUB0REPL00Box385245B00PUBLIC0.pdf (accessed 30 June 2024)

McLaughlin, C.C., & Wyszewianski, L. (2002). Access to care: remembering old lessons. *Health Serv Res*, 37, 1441–1443.

Ministry of Health, Labour and Welfare of Japan (MHLW) (2015). *New Orange Plan*. Tokyo: MHLW. https://www.mhlw.go.jp/file/06-Seisakujouhou-12300000-Roukenkyoku/nop1-2_3.pdf (accessed 13 May 2024)

Ministry of Health, Labour and Welfare of Japan (MHLW) (2016). *Survey of Dental Diseases*. Tokyo: MHLW. https://www.mhlw.go.jp/toukei/list/62-28.html (accessed 30 June 2024).

Ministry of Health, Labour and Welfare of Japan (MHLW) (2017). *Act for Partial Revision of the Long-Term Care Insurance Act, Etc., in Order to Strengthen Long-Term Care Service Infrastructure.* Tokyo: MHLW. https://www.mhlw.go.jp/english/policy/care-welfare/care-welfare-elderly/ (accessed 13 May 2024).

Ministry of Health, Labour and Welfare of Japan (MHLW) (2018). *Manual for Dental Health Check-ups for the Late Elderly* (in Japanese). Tokyo: MHLW. https://www.mhlw.go.jp/content/000410121.pdf (accessed 13 May 2024).

Ministry of Health, Labour and Welfare of Japan (MHLW) (2018b). *Manual for Specific Health Checkups and Specific Health Guidance 2018 version* (in Japanese). Tokyo: MHLW. https://www.mhlw.go.jp/content/10900000/000496784.pdf (accessed 30 June 2024).

Ministry of Health, Labour and Welfare of Japan (MHLW) (2019). *Guidelines for Health Services Based on the Characteristics of Older People*, 2nd edition. Tokyo: MHLW. https://www.mhlw.go.jp/stf/shingi2/0000204952_00001.html (accessed 30 June 2024).

Ministry of Health, Labour and Welfare of Japan (MHLW) (2019b). *The Policy Guidelines for the 2020 Medical Fee Revisions* (in Japanese). Tokyo: MHLW. https://www.mhlw.go.jp/content/12401000/000575290.pdf (accessed 30 June 2024)

Ministry of Health, Labour and Welfare of Japan (MHLW) (2020a). *Comprehensive Survey of Living Conditions in 2019*. Tokyo: MHLW. https://www.mhlw.go.jp/toukei/saikin/hw/k-tyosa/k-tyosa19/index.html (accessed 13 May 2024).

Ministry of Health, Labour and Welfare of Japan (MHLW) (2020b). *Patient Survey* (in Japanese). Tokyo: MHLW. https://www.mhlw.go.jp/toukei/saikin/hw/kanja/20/index.html (accessed 30 June 2024).

Ministry of Health, Labour and Welfare of Japan (MHLW) (2021). *Vital Statistics of Japan 2021*. Tokyo: MHLW. https://www.mhlw.go.jp/toukei/saikin/hw/jinkou/houkoku21/dl/all.pdf (accessed 13 May 2024).

Ministry of Health, Labour and Welfare of Japan (MHLW) (2022a). *Statistics of Medical Care Activities in Public Health Insurance*. Tokyo: MHLW. https://www.mhlw.go.jp/toukei/saikin/hw/sinryo/tyosa21/ (accessed 13 May 2024).

Ministry of Health, Labour and Welfare of Japan (MHLW) (2022b). *Life Tables. List of Statistical Surveys Conducted, 2022*. Tokyo: MHLW. https://www.mhlw.go.jp/toukei/saikin/hw/life/23th/index.html (accessed 13 May 2024).

Ministry of Health, Labour and Welfare of Japan (MHLW) (2022c). *Estimates of National Medical Care Expenditure*. Tokyo: MHLW. https://www.mhlw.go.jp/toukei/saikin/hw/k-iryohi/20/index.html (accessed 13 May 2024).

Ministry of Health, Labour and Welfare of Japan (MHLW) (2022d) *NDB Open Data, 2022*. Tokyo: MHLW. https://www.mhlw.go.jp/stf/seisakunitsuite/bunya/0000177221_00011.html (accessed 13 May 2024).

National Institute of Population and Social Security Research. (2021) *Social Security Expenditure*. https://www.ipss.go.jp/ss-cost/j/fsss-R02/fsss_R02new.html (accessed 13 May 2024).

Ninomiya, T. (2018). Japanese legacy cohort studies: The Hisayama Study. *J Epidemiol*, 28(11), 444–451.

OECD (2019). *Health statistics 2019*. Paris: OECD Publishing.

OECD (2018). *Health at a Glance 2017: OECD Indicators*. Paris: OECD Publishing. https://doi.org/10.1787/health_glance-2017-en (accessed 13 May 2024).

Ozawa, M., Ninomiya, T., Ohara, T. et al. (2013). Dietary patterns and risk of dementia in an elderly Japanese population: the Hisayama Study. *Am J Clin Nutr*, 97(5), 1076–1082.

Reich, M.R., Ikegami, N., Shibuya, K., & Takemi, K. (2011) 50 years of pursuing a healthy society in Japan. *Lancet*, 17, 378(9796), 1051–1053.

Tsuneishi, M., Yamamoto, T., Okumura, Y. et al. (2017). Number of teeth and medical care expenditure. *Health Sci Health Care*, 17, 36–37.

United Nations (2011). *Political Declaration of the High-level Meeting of the General Assembly on the Prevention and Control of Non-communicable Diseases 2011*. https://www.un.org/en/ga/ncdmeeting2011/pdf/NCD_draft_political_declaration.pdf (accessed 13 May 2024).

United Nations (2015) *Transforming Our World: The 2030 Agenda for Sustainable Development*. https://sustainabledevelopment.un.org/content/documents/21252030%20Agenda%20for%20Sustainable%20Development%20web.pdf?_gl=1*1r8pzqb*_ga*MTc0MTMxNjI4MS4xNzE1NjAwNTY5*_ga_TK9BQL5X7Z*MTcxNTYyMzIzMi4xLjAuMTcxNTYyMzIzMi4wLjAuMA (accessed 13 May 2024).

World Health Organization (2010). Health Systems Financing: the Path to Universal Coverage, Geneva: WHO. https://www.who.int/publications/i/item/9789241564021 (accessed 30 June 2024).

World Health Organization (2015). *Tracking Universal Health Coverage: First Global Monitoring Report*. Geneva: WHO. https://www.who.int/publications/i/item/9789241564977 (accessed 13 May 2024).

World Health Organization. (2017). *Tracking Universal Health Coverage: 2017 Global Monitoring Report*. Joint WHO/World Bank Group report. Geneva: WHO. https://www.who.int/publications/i/item/9789241513555 (accessed 13 May 2024).

World Health Organization (2020). *Decade of Healthy Ageing 2020–2030, 73rd World Health Assembly Decisions*. Geneva: WHO. https://www.who.int/news-room/feature-stories/detail/73rd-world-health-assembly-decisions (accessed 13 May 2024).

World Health Organization (2021a). *Decade of Healthy Ageing*. Baseline report. Geneva: WHO. https://cdn.who.int/media/docs/default-source/decade-of-healthy-ageing/decade-proposal-final-apr2020-en.pdf?sfvrsn=b4b75ebc_28 (accessed 13 May 2024).

World Health Organization. (2021b). *Oral Health*. The Seventy-fourth World Health Assembly (WHA74.5). Geneva: WHO. https://apps.who.int/gb/ebwha/pdf_files/WHA74/A74_R5-en.pdf (accessed 13 May 2024).

World Health Organization. (2021c). *UHC Service Coverage Index (SDG 3.8.1)*. Geneva: WHO. https://www.who.int/data/gho/data/indicators/indicator-details/GHO/uhc-index-of-service-coverage (accessed 13 May 2024).

World Health Organization. (2021d). Seventy-fourth World Health Assenbly WHA 74.5 Agenda item 13.2 31 Oral health. Geneva: WHO. https://apps.who.int/gb/ebwha/pdf_files/WHA74/A74_R5-en.pdf (accessed 30 June 2024).

World Health Organization. (2022). *Tracking Universal Health Coverage: 2021 Global Monitoring Report*. Geneva: WHO. https://www.who.int/publications/i/item/9789240040618 (accessed 13 May 2024).

Yoneyama, T., Yoshida, M., Matsui, T., Sasaki, H., and the Oral Care Working Group. (1999). Oral care and pneumonia. *The Lancet*, 354, 515.

Zaitsu, T., Saito, T., Kawaguchi, Y. (2018). The oral healthcare system in Japan. *Healthcare (Basel)*, 6(3), 79.

5

Lessons from the United Kingdom, Europe, North America and Australia

Oral Health for an Ageing Population: Evidence, Policy, Practice and Evaluation, First Edition. Kakuhiro Fukai.
© 2025 John Wiley & Sons Ltd. Published 2025 by John Wiley & Sons Ltd.

5.1 Introduction

Universal health coverage (UHC) is defined as a system in which all people and communities can use the promotive, preventive, curative, rehabilitative and palliative health services they need, whose services are of sufficient quality to be effective, and which ensures that the use of these services does not expose the user to financial hardship [World Health Organization (WHO) 2019a]. This message has been repeatedly reinforced since the 1978 Declaration of Alma-Ata. In 2005, the WHO endorsed UHC as a central goal and stated that health systems must 'be further developed in order to guarantee access to necessary services while providing protection against financial risk' (WHO 2005, 2014). UHC can be understood as a broad legal, rights-based, social humanitarian, health economics and public health concept (Abiiro et al. 2015).

One of the goals of UHC is to create a healthcare system to provide equal accessibility to affordable healthcare for all people. Barriers to healthcare accessibility directly cause deterioration of health, particularly for the elderly and other vulnerable groups. Ageing populations and slow economic growth are prompting most developed nations to reconsider their social security systems, particularly in the area of healthcare reform. Developed countries share some common challenges: how to provide all residents with equal access to a fair, sustainable healthcare system with limited financial resources (Garla et al. 2014; Dror et al. 2016; Eaton et al. 2019; Sinclair 2019).

This chapter reviews the medical health insurance systems of seven developed, Western nations: the UK, Sweden, Australia, Canada, France, Germany and the USA. Japan's system is described in detail in Chapter 4. The characteristics and challenges of these countries' public health insurance systems are summarized based on research reports and government records from 1995 to 2019. Some of these countries have government-funded or social insurance-type systems, while others rely primarily on private insurance. In terms of dental insurance coverage, the developed countries covered in this chapter run the gamut, with some providing government-funded dental insurance, some providing partial coverage, and some relying entirely on private insurance coverage. There is room for improvement in terms of providing dental care to a wider range of people without imposing undue financial burden.

5.2 Medical health insurance systems

Based on funding type, public health insurance systems are mainly divided into three types: (1) the government-funded tax revenue model such as that of the UK, Sweden, Australia and Canada (Table 5.1); (2) the social insurance model, which is financed via compulsory premiums, as in France and Germany (Table 5.2); and (3) the hybrid model, consisting of private insurance for most citizens and the tax revenue model for vulnerable groups, as in the USA (Table 5.3). Japan's system, which is described in detail in Chapter 4, is a social insurance model.

5.2.1 Tax revenue model (government-funded)

5.2.1.1 UK

5.2.1.1.1 Medical insurance system The National Health Service (NHS), established in 1948, provides comprehensive health services, including disease prevention and rehabilitation, for all people. The national government uses national tax revenue to provide medical health services. The system is primarily (> 80%) funded by tax revenue, while over 18% of funding comes from individual contributions (National Health Service premiums).

Table 5.1 Public health insurance systems: tax revenue model.

Country	Insurance system name	Legal basis	Administrative body	Funding sources	Eligibility	Benefits	User charges	Percentage of population covered	Dental health coverage included?
UK	National Health Service (NHS)	The National Health Service Act, 1946	Department of Health	• Tax revenue: 80% or more • Individual premiums: more than 18% • Patient share: more than 1% (costs of outpatient prescription drugs, dental treatments, etc.) • Low-income people have no premium payment obligation	All residents (all adults and children)	• First: see a pre-registered general practitioner (GP). If necessary: the GP introduces patient to specialists in hospitals • Comprehensive health services, including disease prevention, rehabilitation and community health, are provided	• **General medical treatments:** free • **Treatment costs of hospital specialists after GP introduction:** basically free • **Outpatient prescription drugs:** co-payment per prescription • **Eyesight test:** out-of-pocket payment • **Some long-term treatments:** out-of pocket payment • **Exempted from out-of-pocket payments:** persons of age 60 or older, those under age 16, low-income households, pregnant women • **Dental treatments:** basically, NHS covers 80% of costs. – Band 1 dental treatment[1]: £22.7 – Band 2 dental treatment: £62.10 – Band 3 dental treatment: £269.30 (as of April 2019)	100%	Yes

(Continued)

Table 5.1 (Continued)

Country	Insurance system name	Legal basis	Administrative body	Funding sources	Eligibility	Benefits	User charges	Percentage of population covered	Dental health coverage included?
Sweden	–	Hälso-och sjukvårdslag	County councils or municipalities called Landstings[a]	Taxes levied by Landsting (mainly financed through resident and income taxes), and patient co-payments	All residents	Medical treatment provided in kind: outpatient and in-patient care	• **Outpatient care:** fixed co-payment per vist, according to whether first visit or not, age of patient. Free for those under age 20 • **Inpatient care:** fixed co-payment per day, according to age, income. 50–100 krona co-payment per day and free for people under age 18–20 in most Landstings • **Treatment of certain diseases or injuries:** national subsidies provided • **Medical prescriptions:** upper limit is 0.05 times the price of the yearly cap (2200 krona in 2017) • **Dental treatments for people under age 20:** free, covered by Landsting (mainly from resident and income taxes) • **Dental treatments for people of age 20 or more:** partial aids of treatment fees from invalidity insurance	–	Yes

Country	Name	Act	Administered by	Funding	Eligibility	Covered services	Service details	Coverage	
Australia	Medicare	Health Insurance Act, 1973	Federal government	• Medicare levy: 2% of marginal taxable income • Government-funded from general tax revenue: 75%	All residents	• Outpatient care by GPs and medical consultants • Medical prescriptions • Inpatient care and treatment of patients in public hospitals	• **Medical services:** free, including outpatient care by GPs and medical consultants, and medical drugs (prescriptions) • **In-patient care and treatment:** free for Medicare patients in public hospitals • **Out-of-pocket for full amount:** ophthalmology, long-term treatment of chronic diseases, emergency transport • **Dental treatment:** Out-of-pocket for full amount, including orthodontics	100%	No
Canada	Medicare[b]	Canada Health Act, 1984	Provincial and territorial governments	• General tax revenue • State government and block subsidies from federal government	All residents • Canadian nationals • Permanent residents • Immigrants require 3-month waiting period • International students excluded in some provinces	• Inpatient care, medical drugs, outpatient care • Basically out-of-pocket: medical prescriptions, dental treatments, ophthalmology, rehabilitation and nursing care	• **Ophthalmology:** basically out-of-pocket • **Rehabilitation:** basically out-of-pocket • **Nursing care:** basically out-of-pocket • **Dental care:** basically out-of-pocket	100%	No

[a] Landsting: this is the local government of each county, like a state or a province. It mainly provides medical services, such as establishing and managing medical facilities. Medical staff, such as doctors and nurses, work as a public servants for their Landsting. Basically, the costs are covered by the tax revenue of the Landsting, mainly from resident and income taxes, as well as patient co-payment.

[b] Medical care system in Canada consists of two kinds of doctors: GPs and medical specialists. First, a patient sees a GP. After that, if necessary, the GP introduces the patient to a hospital specialist. A patient cannot see a specialist without an introduction from a GP.

Table 5.2 Public health insurance systems: social insurance model.

Country	Insurance system name	Legal basis	Administrative body	Funding sources	Eligibility	Benefits	User Charges	Percentage of population covered	Dental health coverage included?
France	General Health Care Fund Mainly consists of workers in commerce and industry	Social security code	CNAMTS: Caisse Nationale de l'Assurance Maladie des Travailleurs Salariés	1) **Premiums** • Based on gross earnings: • 0.75% levied on employees • 12.89% levied on employers 2) **Public share** • 36% share of the employees as general social contribution (CSG) • 15.2% from earmarked taxes imposed on tobacco and alcohol • 1.5% from state subsidies • 44.5% from health insurance premiums (2016)	Everyone must join a compulsory health insurance system, according to their occupation. 1) **Systems for employees by occupation:** • General system: for employees in commerce and industry (92% of the population) • Separate systems for civil servants, local public officials, Paris Travel Bureau, sailors, and soldiers 2) **Systems for non-employees**: self-employed, priests	• Basically a reimbursement model • Hospitalization: directly paid to medical institutions	• **Outpatient care:** 70% • **In-patient care:** 80% • **General medical drugs:** basically 65% • **Most user charges:** covered by benevolent association and mutual benefit association. The remainder is out of pocket. • **Dental treatments:**[a] 70% reimbursed by the state if covered by French Social Security (Carte Vital) Orthodontics: not covered under the state system.	61.5 million (92% of all residents)	Yes

Germany	Statutory Health Insurance (Gesetzliche Krankenversicherung)	SGBV	Sick Funds	• General insurance premium rate is 14.6%: half is paid by employer, and half by employee • Additional insurance premium:[b] 1.1% levied on insured person (estimated average in 2017) • State subsidy	• Employees whose income is below a certain level; self-employed traders in agriculture and forestry • Not compulsory for employees with incomes above a certain level, as well as the self-employed and public servants. Basically, those who are not eligible for a Sick Fund are required to join national health insurance or private health insurance	• Basically, payment in kind: – Medical allowance – Preventive care allowance – Medical rehabilitation allowance – Home nursing allowance • Cash payment: invalidity benefit	• **Outpatient care:** free from 2013 • **In-patient care:** 10 euro per day; maximum 28 days per year • **Medical drugs:** 10% of the price (minimum 5 euro, maximum 10 euro) • **Dental treatment for people age 18 or older:** normal insurance benefits plus additional benefits according to the choice of the insured. • **Dental treatment for persons under 18:** the sick funds provide full reimbursement for surgical dental treatment and necessary orthodontic care, and certain prophylactic treatments are provided free of charge	87% of all residents (2018)	Yes

[a] Dental treatments in France: normally the patient is charged the full amount for the treatment, and then 70% is reimbursed for adults (100% for children aged 6–18).

[b] Additional insurance premium: the insurance premiums are collected in the medical fund and then divided into separate subsidies for each disease category. Additional insurance premiums are levied for disease categories that are difficult to cover with subsidies from the medical fund. To avoid overburdening low-income residents, those for whom the additional premium is 2% or more of their income can receive a subsidy.

Table 5.3 Public health insurance systems: mixed model (tax revenue and social insurance model).

Country	Insurance System Name	Legal Basis	Administrative Body	Funding Sources	Eligibility	Benefits	User Charges	Percentage of Population Covered	Dental Health Coverage Included?
USA	Medicare[1] (Social Insurance Model)	Social Security Act 18	Department of Health and Human Services Centers for Medicare and Medicaid Services (CMS) (Part A and B) Private Insurance (Parts C and D)	**Part A:** social security tax on employees (divided fifty-fifty between employers and employees; full amount paid by the self-employed) **Part B:** monthly payments of $134–428.60, levied on individuals according to annual income **Part C, D:** depending on each plan The National Treasury covers the balance of payments for private insurance premiums	Individuals age 65 and older Individuals under 65 with disabilities Individuals with end-stage renal disease (permanent kidney failure that requires dialysis or transplant)	**Part A:** (Hospital Insurance) Compulsory insurance that covers inpatient care and advanced nursing care **Part B:** (Medical Insurance) Voluntary insurance that covers outpatient care **Part C:** (Medicare Advantage) Voluntary insurance for those already enrolled in Part A and B, providing coverage equal or greater than that included under Part A and B. **Part D:** (Medicare Prescription Drug Plans) Voluntary insurance covering prescription drug costs for outpatient care	• **Inpatient care (Part A):** $1,340 deductible per hospitalization – No charge for 1–60 days of hospitalization – $335 out-of-pocket per day for 61st–90th days of hospitalization – $670 out-of-pocket per day beyond 90 days of hospitalization • **Outpatient care (Part B):** Annual $183 deductible – 20% out-of-pocket for amounts beyond the deductible • **Medicare Advantage Plan (Part C):** extra benefits such as routine dental, routine vision, prescription drug coverage • **Part C and D:** depending on each plan • **Dental coverage:** No coverage for routine dental work such as dental exams, cleanings, fillings, crowns, bridges and dentures under Original Medicare (Part A and B) Some exceptions: medical reconstruction required due to accident-related jaw damage, treatment for jaw-related diseases, and tooth extractions directly caused by a disease	55.62 million (17.2%) (2017)	No Some exceptions

| Medicaid (Tax Revenue Model) | Social Security Act 19 | Department of Health and Human Services Centers for Medicare and Medicaid Services (CMS) Management: each state | • No premiums • Federal and state governments share the costs. | • Low-income adults and children • Pregnant women • People with disabilities | • Regular medical services: inpatient care and medical services • Long-term nursing care | • **Dental coverage for children under the age of 21:** – pain relief and infection treatment – tooth restoration – dental health maintenance – any service determined to be medically necessary • **Dental coverage for adults over the age of 21:** varies by state | 62.49 million (19.3%) (2017) | Yes |

[1] The United States has not achieved universal health coverage. The medical health system relies heavily on private insurance. Around 60% of Americans are covered by employer-provided private medical insurance.

Except for emergency care, patients see a licensed general practitioner (GP) first. The GP can then refer patients to hospital consultants if deemed necessary. Medical treatments funded by private insurance or individuals represent only around 1% of the national health expenditure [Tinker 2003; Fukuda et al. 2009; Steele 2009; Ministry of Health, Labour and Welfare (MHLW) of Japan 2018]. GPs are reimbursed based on a per-capita payment system (according to the number of registered patients). The system is designed to incentivise disease prevention: if a GP's registered patients maintain good health through preventive activities, health service consumption will be reduced. As the income of the GP remains unchanged, GPs are motivated to implement preventive activities, which is expected to have a positive effect on public health (Fukuda et al. 2009).

General medical treatments are free of charge for all residents who have pre-registered with their own GP. In most cases, patients can see hospital specialists at no charge if introduced by their GP.

Prescription drugs for outpatients are charged at a fixed rate per prescription. Patients themselves bear the full cost of eyesight tests and some long-term treatments. People aged 60 or over, those under 16, those from low-income households, and pregnant women are exempted from those payments (Tinker 2003; Fukuda et al. 2009; Steele 2009; MHLW of Japan 2018).

5.2.1.1.2 Dental insurance system The NHS covers approximately 80% of dental treatment expenses. There are three bands of fixed rate charges for dental treatments, plus a special rate for urgent treatment. As of 2024, the dental treatment fees are as follows (NHS 2024):

- Band 1 (£26.80) – examinations, X-rays, scaling and polishing, preventive treatments, adjusting false teeth, treating sensitive cementum.
- Band 2 (£73.50) – treatments in band 1 plus restorations, root canal treatments, extractions, oral surgeries, and scaling and root planing.
- Band 3 (£319.10) – Treatments in bands 1 and 2 plus crowns, bridges, dentures, inlays/onlays and orthodontic treatments/appliances.
- Urgent (£26.80) – emergency treatment and pain relief.

Treatments such as veneers and braces are only available in the NHS if there is a clinical need for them (not for cosmetic reasons). Similarly, other cosmetic treatments, such as tooth whitening, are not available in the NHS (Tinker 2003; Fukuda et al. 2009; Steele 2009; Kravitz et al. 2015; MHLW of Japan 2018).

5.2.1.2 Sweden

5.2.1.2.1 Medical insurance system Sweden has a universal healthcare system that is primarily government-funded but decentralized: county councils and municipal governments are responsible for providing services (Fukuda et al. 2009; Kravitz et al. 2015; Berglund et al 2017; MHLW of Japan 2018). Most healthcare is funded by the national social insurance system. The Swedish healthcare system is mainly financed by taxes levied by county councils and municipalities, as well as patient fees. County councils regulate medical prices and services provided at the local level.

Public coverage is extensive, so the burden on individual patients is very small, capped at 1100 krona per year in 2017. Swedish residents do not have to pay more than 300 krona for each primary care doctor visit. Free outpatient services are provided for residents under the age of 20, and in-patient services are free for those under 18 or 20 in most counties. Fixed co-payment is set for outpatient care depending on whether it is the first visit or not, the age of the patient and the treatment destination. Fixed co-payment per day is set for in-patient care depending on age, income and hospitalizations of patients. Prescription drugs are not free, but individual drug expenses are capped at 2200 krona per year. The government covers expenses that exceed this amount. Pharmacies are connected to a centralized data system that stores the medical history of each patient and makes it available to all pharmacies (MHLW of Japan 2018).

More attention is given to healthcare at the local government level than at the national level, because local governments have fewer other responsibilities demanding their attention. However, movement of the working population from rural to urban areas has led to regional disparities and unfairness in access to healthcare resources. This is a challenge that needs to be addressed by the government (Fukuda et al. 2009).

5.2.1.2.2 Dental insurance system   Oral healthcare is the responsibility of county governments, but counties are not required to provide the services themselves. Dental care is not included in the general health care system, but is partly subsidized by the government.

Dental care for children and adolescents (Osterberg et al. 1995; Biggs 2012; Molarius et al. 2014; Kravitz et al. 2015; Berglund et al. 2017; MHLW of Japan 2018) is free of charge up to the age of 19. Some county councils have extended dental care provisions to include young people over 20. Care is provided on a regular basis and is individually targeted. Children up to the age of 19 are assigned to a particular dentist for regular care and treatment. Dental care is financed and provided through the counties and carried out either by dentists within the Public Dental Service (PDS) or by private practitioners (PPs). Most dental care for children and adolescents is carried out within the PDS.

Dental care for adults (Osterberg et al. 1995; Biggs 2012; Molarius et al. 2014; Kravitz et al. 2015; Berglund et al. 2017; MHLW of Japan 2018) is provided by dentists from both PDS and PPs. Adults pay nearly the full amount of their own dental fees up front, but the social insurance system reimburses a portion of the cost for most dental care.

An annual dental care voucher or dental grant of €15 is given to all residents aged 30–74. For those aged 20–29 and 75 or older, the voucher is €30 per year. Not all kinds of dental care are reimbursable, however. Rather, preventive care and disease treatment are prioritized. Unused vouchers can be accumulated and used for a period of up to two years.

5.2.1.3 Australia

5.2.1.3.1 Medical insurance system   Australia has a universal healthcare system that covers primary care and is administered by GPs, similar to the UK. It has been mainly funded by Medicare since 1984. Healthcare is delivered by both government (national, state and local) and private insurance providers, which are in turn covered by Medicare (Anderson et al. 1998; Roberts-Thomson and Stewart 2003; Anikeeva et al. 2013; Brennan et al. 2013; Teusner et al. 2014; Teusner et al. 2015; Gnanamanickam et al. 2018; JASIC Inc 2019). Medicare itself is funded by a Medicare levy, which is a 2% levy on residents' taxable income over a certain amount. Higher income earners pay an additional 1–1.5% levy called a Medicare Levy Surcharge if they do not have private insurance. Residents with certain medical conditions, foreign residents and low-income earners are exempt from paying the levy.

The federal government-administered Medicare insurance scheme covers the majority of primary health service expenses. It also covers a portion of outpatient care expenses and all in-patient care expenses.

5.2.1.3.2 Dental insurance system   Australians must pay out of pocket for dental care services, including orthodontics, unless they hold a Health Care card, which may entitle them to subsidized access (JASIC Inc 2019).

5.2.1.4 Canada

5.2.1.4.1 Medical insurance system Medical care in Canada is delivered through provincial and territorial-funded Medicare systems. All eligible residents can access in-patient and outpatient medical care through this system (Bhatti 2007; Duncan 2014; Thompson et al. 2014; Morgan et al. 2017; MHLW of Japan 2018; Tuohy 2018; Zivkovic et al. 2020). It provides coverage for 70% of healthcare needs. The remaining 30%, including prescription drugs, optometry and rehabilitation, is paid for by patients themselves.

5.2.1.4.2 Dental insurance system Dental care is not covered by public medical insurance, based on the Canada Health Act of 1984. Approximately 60% of dental care expenses are covered by employment-based insurance, and 35% are out of pocket. Dental care and regular check-ups are therefore only accessible to those who can afford to pay the fees (Bhatti 2007; Duncan 2014. Thompson et al. 2014; MHLW of Japan 2018).

5.2.2 Social insurance model (funded via compulsory premiums)

5.2.2.1 France

5.2.2.1.1 Medical insurance system Healthcare in France is considered to be a fundamental human right for all residents, thereby obligating the government to provide universal access. The French healthcare system has provided UHC since 2000, delivered via two basic routes: health insurance is provided to anyone who has stable and regular employment, and free coverage is also provided to disadvantaged people via a fee exemption system.

The French healthcare system is funded via a social insurance model with the premiums based on income, as in Table 5.2 (Kravitz et al. 2015; MHLW of Japan 2018; Mercier et al. 2019). This system is funded in part by compulsory health contributions levied on all employee salaries, paid by both employers and employees, and in part by central government funding. The state has also been increasingly involved in controlling health expenditures covered by a separate statutory health insurance system, which is funded by employer and employee payroll taxes, taxes levied on tobacco and alcohol, and state subsidies.

All legal residents are legally required to join the system according to their occupation, which is administered by a health insurance management system called Caisse Primaire d'Assurance Maladie (or simply 'Caisse'). The system differs by occupation as follows:

1) Systems for employees include a general system, to which 92% of employees are registered, including those involved in commerce and industry. Separate systems are administered for civil servants, local public officials, the Paris Travel Bureau, sailors and soldiers.
2) Systems for non-employees include those for the self-employed and for priests.

Insurance benefits are delivered via reimbursement, except for hospitalization, in which case the reimbursement is issued directly to medical institutions. Patients are required to pay out-of-pocket for 70% of outpatient care expenses, 80% of in-patient care expenses, and 65% of medication expenses. However, most of these expenses are actually covered by benevolent association and mutual benefit associations. The remainder is a final self-payment.

5.2.2.1.2 Dental insurance system Citizens can claim reimbursement of 70% of the dental care fees from the state if they are covered by the French Social Security system, called Carte Vital. Normally, patients are charged the full amount for treatments up front, and then 70% of the expenses for most dental treatments are reimbursed for adults and 100% for children. Orthodontic treatment is not covered under the state system. Basic dental care, including consultations, treatment of cavities and tooth extractions, is covered by the state, but more complex or cosmetic treatments such as tooth whitening and implants are usually paid for by patients themselves or via private insurance plans. However, from 2021, dental prostheses have been fully reimbursed (Pegon-Machat et al. 2016; Mazevet et al. 2018).

Children are offered free dental check-ups every 3 years between the ages of 6 and 18. Families with children receive a letter from the Caisse, which entitles children to receive an examination by a dentist free of charge (Kravitz et al. 2015; MHLW of Japan 2018).

5.2.2.2 Germany

5.2.2.2.1 Medical insurance system   Germany has a UHC system paid for by a combination of public health insurance (*Gesetzliche Krankenversicherung*) and private health insurance (*Private Krankenversicherung*), a system that dates back to the 1880s (Kravitz et al. 2015; Ziller et al. 2015; Bock et al. 2016, 2017; MHLW of Japan 2018). It is a legal obligation for anyone living in Germany to have public or private health insurance. The majority of people are enrolled in public health insurance. Salaried workers and employees with a yearly income below 60 750 euros (2019) are automatically enrolled into one of 130 public non-profit 'sick funds' at common rates for all members.

Salaried workers and employees with a yearly income above 60 750 euros (2019), as well as students, civil servants and self-employed workers, can choose whether to enrol in public health insurance or to opt for private health insurance, where their contribution is based on risk assessment formulas.

5.2.2.2.2 Dental insurance system   Dental fees, whether covered by the sick funds or by private insurance, are regulated by the government. The sick funds provide full reimbursement for dental treatment and necessary orthodontic treatment for people under the age of 18. Those under 18 are also eligible to receive certain prophylactic treatments free of charge. Traditionally, public health insurance has not covered dental care for adults. In 2004, public insurance coverage for dental care was introduced for adults aged 18 years and over. For dental treatments exceeding the pre-defined range of necessary care, such as dental prostheses, insured people are required to make co-payments.

Before seeking general care via the public health system, a patient must obtain a voucher from the sick fund. This voucher serves as both proof of entitlement to care and the dentist's claim form for reimbursement of the fee-for-service (Kravitz et al. 2015).

5.2.3   Mixed model (tax revenue and social insurance model) (government and insurer-funded)

5.2.3.1   USA

The USA has no universal public health insurance system. For most residents, private health insurance is provided by employers as an employment benefit. However, there is a public health insurance system that provides coverage for specific groups of people: elderly people aged 65 years and over, and low earners who meet certain eligibility requirements. In this section, I describe these three types of insurance coverage that make up the health insurance system of the US.

5.2.3.1.1 Medical insurance system   Health insurance in the USA includes private insurance, social insurance programmes such as Medicare, and social welfare programmes like Medicaid and the Children's Health Insurance Program (CHIP), as detailed in Table 5.3 (MHLW of Japan 2018;

Masters 2022; NY Health Access). Public health insurance is the primary source of coverage for most seniors as well as low-income children and their families.

Medicare provides health insurance for seniors aged 65 and over, as well as totally or permanently disabled individuals and people with end-stage renal disease and amyotrophic lateral sclerosis. Medicare requires considerable cost-sharing, so 90% of Medicare enrolees have supplemental health insurance.

Medicaid, which was instituted in 1965, is a social welfare or social protection programme which provides coverage for people who cannot afford private health insurance. It is funded jointly by the federal and state governments, and it is administered at the state level. CHIP is a federal–state partnership to provide health insurance for certain children and their families who do not qualify for Medicaid but cannot afford private insurance (Steinmo and Watts 1995; Ross 2002; Schrimshaw et al. 2011; Manski et al. 2014; Manski et al. 2015; Blackwell et al. 2019; Willink 2019).

5.2.3.1.2 *Dental insurance system* Original Medicare (Part A and B) does not cover routine dental care such as dental exams, cleanings, fillings, crowns, bridges and dentures (Masters 2022). Some exceptions are medical reconstruction of the jaw after an accident that causes jaw damage, diseases involving the jaw, and tooth extraction in cases where the need for the extraction arises as a direct result of a serious disease. Medicare Advantage Plans, which are offered by private insurers but must be approved by Medicare, cover additional dental services such as:

- Cleanings
- Exams
- X-rays
- Diagnostic services
- Restorative services (fillings)
- Root canal treatment
- Periodontal disease treatment
- Extractions
- Crowns, bridges, implants, and dentures.

Dental coverage under Medicaid is extremely limited, including only essential services (Haney 2022). Children under the age of 21 are eligible for Medicaid's Early Periodic Screening, Diagnosis and Treatment (EPSDT) programme. Under this programme, children can receive periodic oral evaluations, routine preventive dental care every 6 months, and restorative and emergency dental care.

There is also a Medicaid Orthodontic Benefits programme for children under 21 years old with severe malocclusions causing functional impairment. The coverage is limited to 3 years of treatment and 1 year of retention care.

The services covered under Medicaid for adults over the age of 21 vary by state (Haney 2022). Services normally covered include preventive dental care such as check-ups, oral exams, cleaning, X-rays and sealants; restorative services such as crowns, dentures and orthodontic braces to treat injuries, temporomandibular joint (TMJ) treatment or sleep apnoea; root canal treatments and oral surgery; and other types of dental work considered medically necessary. Medicaid rarely covers dental implant expenses in full. It also does not cover cosmetic dental procedures for adults under any circumstances.

5.2.4 Discussion

The government-funded tax revenue model, such as that in the UK, makes it relatively easy to control the overall healthcare costs of a nation (WHO 2004; Fukuda et al. 2009). However, this model is always accompanied by quality and efficiency problems such as long waiting times for treatment and hospitalization. The countries covered in this chapter do not provide adequate funding for dental coverage for their residents: some place nearly all of the financial burden on patients themselves, while others are partially funded by the government. Due to a shortage of dentists in public healthcare systems, long waiting times and heavy financial burdens for dental treatment often motivate patients to travel to other countries to receive cross-border healthcare (Fukuda et al. 2009; Footman et al. 2014). For example, the EU member states are confronting serious problems related to the free movement of patients and healthcare professionals across national borders (Fukuda et al. 2009). Decisions regarding health insurance coverage must be discussed and negotiated between and among countries, across entire regions and even at the global level.

In the insurer-funded social insurance model, such as that of France, it is more difficult to control increasing medical costs because it is a fee-for-service system funded by compulsory premiums. This means that increases in medical expenses are compensated for by increasing health insurance premiums. This has a negative effect on the national economy itself, because it reduces the purchasing power and motivation of residents (Saltman et al. 2004; Fukuda et al. 2009).

Finally, there is the special case of the US, where public health insurance covers only a limited portion of the population: most seniors aged 65 years and over, and low-income children and their families. The US needs to reform and enlarge its public healthcare system in order to ensure that all people receive fair access to well-funded, high-quality health care services.

5.3 Long-term care system

5.3.1 Background

As the global population ages, older people more often need the care and support of others as they experience significant loss of their intrinsic capacity and functional abilities. It is not surprising, therefore, that long-term care (LTC) is the fastest developing policy area in Europe, the USA and other high-income countries. However, few countries have positioned dental and oral health services as integral to their national LTC systems.

Governance and funding mechanisms for LTC provisions vary from country to country. This section therefore describes the current situation of LTC provisions, focusing on funding sources, in some of the countries whose insurance systems have been described earlier in this chapter.

Common approaches and challenges can be identified in how countries have begun providing LTC to their rapidly ageing populations, even though the funding and service delivery mechanisms may be different (Joshua 2017).

First, many countries have been shifting away from providing LTC in residential settings and towards enabling people to age in place, which is often accompanied by giving them more freedom to choose their care provider. At the same time, countries are distributing funds from central governments to the local government level in an effort to reduce disparities in service provision, and establishing publicly funded LTC systems, whether funded by a social insurance system such as in Germany, Japan and the USA (Medicare) or a tax-based system such as in the UK and Scandinavia.

The traditional approach to medical care for older people has been to focus on symptoms and disease, with diagnosis, treatment and management being the main focus. However, focusing too much on disease diagnosis and treatment overlooks the natural decline in intrinsic capacity – both cognitive and physical functions – which accompany ageing. Shifting the focus to functional decline rather than disease involves national, regional or community screening programmes using standardized assessment tools to improve early detection of functional decline and provide advice regarding possible care and management options. It would also require the implementation of training programmes for LTC providers as well as educational programmes for family and other informal caregivers. Such programmes need to be implemented as part of a comprehensive and integrated community-based approach characterized by multidisciplinary cooperation (WHO 2019b) (Figure 5.1).

Although these approaches to improving LTC in ageing societies are both desirable and supported by the evidence, implementing them requires careful consideration of long-term funding and sustainability, which is a major challenge for all countries. In ageing countries with well-developed social welfare systems, working-age adults are already struggling to save for their own retirement while shouldering heavy tax burdens to support older people, so most countries are ill equipped to cover the costs that will be required to implement comprehensive LTC systems. This means that when countries implement LTC systems, they must make efforts to limit the growth of LTC expenditure over time in order to make such programmes sustainable. This is most often done by limiting the provision of such services to those who are deemed to be most in need of care.

5.3.2 UK

In the UK, the NHS covers LTC in the community and in nursing homes. Non-medical LTC is provided by local social services departments on a means-tested basis, with the exception of Scotland, which provides universal LTC. In the UK, LTC funding comes mainly from the central government, but also partly from local taxes and user fees. Since the 1980s, as long-term hospitalization declined and use of residential care services and nursing homes increased, LTC services moved from being free at the point of provision to a system of means-testing and being funded in part by user fees (Joshua 2017).

Policy developments, particularly in England, have sought to promote cross-boundary collaboration between medical care and LTC (also known as 'adult social care' in the UK), mainly at the local level, through the introduction of primary care trusts (publicly owned entities with a certain degree of independence from the NHS itself), pooled budgets and joint appointments. The Health and Social Care Act 2012 provided for wide-ranging reform of the health system in England.

Long-term care is financed both from central government block grants and from locally-sourced revenue raised through local taxes and user fees. While both are considered important components of LTC, medical care and social care are distinct, with the former providing universal healthcare and the latter providing non-medical care. The latter provides a means-tested 'safety net' mechanism for people with low incomes and few assets. Health services (under the Ministry of Health) are funded by central tax revenues and National Insurance contributions (NICs), while the main provider of LTC is local government, whose policies are set by the Ministry of Health.

Local government cannot contribute towards the cost of long-term care and support in a care home if the adult has assets above a certain level. The Means Testing Scheme is a system whereby fees are based on ability to pay. For people receiving state support in residential care homes, local

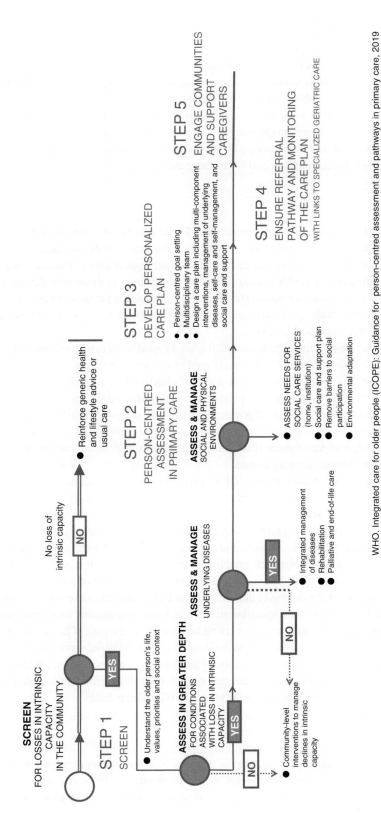

Figure 5.1 Generic care pathway: person-centred assessment and pathways in primary care. *Source:* WHO (2019b).

authorities collect all income (including pensions and benefits) except for a minimum weekly personal allowance. Older people receiving LTC in their own homes are usually required to pay a fee unless their net income is below a certain level, which is determined by national eligibility criteria. The national eligibility criteria take into consideration not what needs an individual has, but whether the person is unable to perform certain activities of daily living (ADLs) and whether this has a significant impact on the person's well-being. Local authorities can then set their own needs eligibility thresholds based on the national criteria. This process ensures that if a person has eligible needs, a care plan can be developed with their input to meet the outcomes they want to achieve (Joshua 2017; Karagiannidou and Wittenberg 2022).

5.3.3 Germany

Until the launch of the Long-term Care Insurance (LTCI) Act in 1994, Germany did not have a comprehensive public system to fund LTC. Previously, older dependents and their families had to pay out-of-pocket if they needed access to formal LTC services. Publicly funded, means-tested social assistance through the health insurance system was limited to those who did not have sufficient resources to meet their care needs. However, social insurance provided under the LTCI Act, along with mandatory private LTCI have made the German LTC system comprehensive, covering nearly the entire population (Joshua 2017).

Germany has taken important steps to establish a solid financial structure to ensure the sustainability of their LTC, thereby providing adequate guarantees for its citizens. The national government is responsible for providing an efficient and cost-effective LTC infrastructure and ensuring that the scale of services provided is appropriate, as well as ensuring the quality and efficiency of LTC facilities. It is the task of all levels of government (federal, state and local) to eliminate gaps in the provision of services and to ensure consistent access to LTC in the various regions of Germany. This includes bearing both investment (such as construction subsidies) and maintenance costs of all local, state and non-profit nursing homes.

The version of the LTCI system introduced in 2016 focuses on ADLs and instrumental ADLs (IADLs), but also takes into account physical, mental and psychological disabilities, with an emphasis on maintaining independence, which is linked to five care-requirement levels. Eligibility is determined by a medical review board, which assesses independence in the following six areas: mobility, cognitive and communication skills, behavioural and psychological problems, ability to care for oneself, needs related to existing illnesses and ongoing treatments, daily routines and social contacts. A comprehensive assessment is made by assigning different weights to each of these indicators.

This approach measures the degree of dependence on LTC rather than the time or frequency of support required. LTCI benefits are specified in the LTCI Act, and eligible recipients can choose between home care, day care, night care or nursing home care. In the case of home care, recipients can choose between cash benefits (of lower value) and in-kind specialized services (of almost twice the value), or a combination of the two. Benefits for institutionalized residents are higher than that of in-kind services for home residents. Under this system, the value of the LTC benefit is linked to the recipient's level of dependence (Karagiannidou and Wittenberg 2022).

5.3.4 France

In France, LTC for the elderly and disabled is situated in a specific sector of the social system referred to as the 'health and social care sector' or the 'third sector'. This sector is divided into two sub-sectors: care for older people and care for disabled people. Care is provided in private residences or elderly care homes. In addition, intermediate care services provide temporary care for dependent patients and respite services for carers. There are also benefits provided for frail older people to hire caregivers, a large private insurance sector and an active informal carer network.

In 2004, the Caisse Nationale de Solidarité pour l'Autonomie (CNSA) was established to fund, plan and coordinate LTC at the national level. Under this system, LTC costs related to medical and nursing services provided at home or in institutions are funded via social health insurance. On the other hand, social care related to dependency (i.e. costs outside the scope of health insurance) is covered under two separate schemes:

1) For the dependent elderly, Allocation Personnalisée d'Autonomie (APA) partially covers the costs of an 'assistance plan' based on assessed need and income.
2) For disabled persons under 60 years of age, Prestation de Compensation de Handicap (PCH) covers LTC services.

In addition to APA and PCH, France has a large LTC insurance market. The French LTC insurance system is a flat-rate payment system, which allows policyholders to choose the care and services they want. Compensation insurance is the predominant type of insurance in France. The basic private coverage offered by private LTC insurance schemes is marketed as a complement to the limited public benefits offered by APA and PCH. In 2013, an additional tax (Additional Solidarity Contribution for Autonomy, or CASA) was levied on pensioners' income, strengthening the LTC funding base. Then, in 2014, the monthly cap on LTC benefits was raised and respite care for informal caregivers was included (Joshua 2017).

5.3.5 Sweden

Sweden pursues the general goal of providing LTC services free of charge to all who need them, regardless of their economic situation. Traditionally, LTC was provided almost exclusively by families; however, beginning in the 1940s, publicly funded LTC has evolved in order to implement a more universal approach, providing for the poor and the elderly.

In Sweden, municipalities are responsible for financing and providing LTC. The cost is covered by general income tax, the majority of which is local income tax, as well as user fees. The national government, on the other hand, is responsible for overall oversight and for establishing the general legal and financial framework for healthcare and social security, including LTC services for the elderly. The state also provides special grants for the purpose of healthcare for the elderly. There are equalization grants aimed at redistributing revenues between local governments to reduce regional disparities in LTC for the elderly.

Around 90% of care services are provided directly by local governments, with a small amount outsourced to the private sector. In certain regions, a 'client choice system' has been adopted, whereby users can choose their service provider. The goal of care services is to enable people to live an active life in old age and to be able to determine their own daily activities. In Sweden, the emphasis is on independence, which means that home care services and 'special housing' are provided to ensure that people can live independently and safely into old age. In order to give older people the right to receive good-quality medical and social care while maintaining their dignity, independent of their financial situation, the Social Services Act was established and care services are provided in accordance with this Act. The responsibility for the operation of long-term care services lies with the municipalities and, in principle, LTC services are provided according to the needs and circumstances of each person.

Care services are provided on the basis of an application by individuals or their families, after which a needs assessor determines the level of care required and the type of services to be provided. There is no standardized classification of level of care required; rather, the assessment and determination criteria differ by municipality. Care services include home-based services (home help services, day services, short stays, home nursing, meal delivery services, safety alarms, home modification, transport services, etc.) and institutional services. The three types of institutions available are 'service houses' (housing complexes for the elderly), 'nursing homes' (for those in need of serious nursing care), and 'group homes' (for those with dementia) (Joshua 2017; Karagiannidou and Wittenberg 2022).

5.3.6 USA

In the USA, individual responsibility for LTC has traditionally been emphasized, as reflected in the modest safety net provided by Medicare and Medicaid only for those most in need of LTC.

Medicare is a federally administered health insurance scheme for people aged 65 and over, people with physical disabilities and people with severe kidney impairment requiring dialysis or transplantation. Medicare covers a limited amount of LTC, including care in a nursing home after a period in hospital of more than 3 days.

Medicaid is not a social insurance scheme but rather a joint federal and state programme based on means testing and need, covering healthcare and LTC costs for the poor. However, due to high LTC costs, nearly 65% of nursing home residents are Medicaid recipients.

Most people with dual eligibility for Medicare and Medicaid are disabled, and Medicare serves as the primary payer for a range of services for people with dual eligibility. Medicaid provides cost-sharing assistance and may pay for services that are not covered or only partially covered by Medicare.

The Home- and Community-Based Service (HCBS) programme was introduced in 1995 to correct Medicaid's bias towards residential provision. In some states, Medicaid can pay for home-based services, assisted living or residential care, or nursing home care for eligible individuals. To qualify for Medicaid, a person must ensure that they no longer have savings or other assets to pay for services. This was introduced under the Affordable Care Act (ACA).

In 2010, the HCBS programme was developed and expanded as a replacement for institutional care. Many states are expanding HCBS, but the bias towards care in nursing homes persists. The reason for this is that insurance coverage for nursing homes is mandatory, while other components of HCBS programmes are voluntary. To encourage community-based LTC services, the federal government began providing additional support to transition people from nursing homes to the community through the Nursing Home Conversion Programme and the Money Follows the Person (MFP) grant introduced in 2006.

Long-term services and support are financed from both private and public sources, but the majority are covered by publicly funded health insurance schemes. There are few affordable options in the private insurance market, and Medicare coverage is limited, so people who do not have sufficient financial resources typically turn to Medicaid.

The HCBS programmes account for the majority of Medicaid LTC spending. However, it should be noted that the majority of LTC still consists of informal, unpaid assistance by spouses and other relatives, and the cost of LTC often exceeds what individuals and families can afford when other personal and household expenses are considered. Facilities such as nursing homes and residential care homes are the most expensive element of such care: in 2015, nursing homes cost between USD 50 000 and USD 280 000 per year, while assisted living facilities cost between USD 30 000 and USD 94 000.

In general, HCBS is cheaper than facility-based LTC, but it can still represent a significant financial burden for individuals and their families. Older people seeking to hedge the risk of needing expensive LTC services can take out private insurance. Private LTC insurance is generally not available to all people who need LTC now or in the future, due to high premiums. Although private LTC insurance started as nursing home insurance and has been available for about 30 years, the market for this insurance product is relatively small.

Medicaid policy has traditionally directed people with LTC needs to institutions, but most recipients prefer to continue to live at home or in the community while receiving services. The HCBS programme enables many people to live at home and generally provides assistance with LTC needs as assessed by the number of ADLs (essential activities such as bathing, dressing, moving from bed to chair, eating, and using the toilet) and IADLs (activities needed for independent living such as shopping and answering the phone) that a person cannot perform on their own. In 2015, an estimated 10 million people aged 65 and over lived in the community with ADL or IADL disabilities. A further estimated 6.5 million people aged 65 and over lived in nursing homes (Joshua 2017; Karagiannidou and Wittenberg 2022; Angrisani et al. 2022).

5.4 Conclusion

Dental care is not covered or only partially covered in most of the developed nations discussed in this chapter, even though dental treatments often impose a heavy financial burden on patients. Public health insurance in the USA only serves as the primary source of coverage for people in a specific age group and those who have certain socioeconomic characteristics. There is potential for improvement so that a wider range of people can receive higher-quality public health care with reduced financial burden.

In Europe and the USA, where super-ageing societies are on the rise, the demand for LTC is increasing in all countries. In this context, the common challenge that all countries face is to limit the growth of LTC expenditure in order to make programmes to support older people sustainable. In the USA and Europe, the solution so far has generally taken the form of limiting the provision of targeted services to those deemed to be most in need of care.

At the same time, LTC systems play an important role in preventing the worsening of health conditions of people requiring LTC, thereby extending the healthy longevity of older people while allowing them to remain in their own communities. The traditional approach to healthcare for older people was characterized by a narrow focus on disease diagnosis and treatment, overlooking the decline in intrinsic capacity – cognitive and physical function – that accompanies ageing. The challenge moving forward will be to develop a comprehensive, community-based approach, with the government providing guidelines for standardized assessment and response to functional decline, including improving the training of LTC providers.

References

Abiiro, G.A. & de Allegri, M. (2015). Universal health coverage from multiple perspectives: a synthesis of conceptual literature and global debates. *BMC Int Health Hum Rights*, 15, 17.

Anderson, R., Treasure, E.T., Whitehouse, N.H. (1998). Oral health systems in Europe. Part I: Finance and entitlement to care. *Commun Dent Health*, 15(3), 145–149.

Angrisani, M., Regalado, J.C.O., Hashiguchi T.C.O. (2022). Financial social protection and individual out-of-pocket costs of long-term care in the USA and Europe: An observational study. *EClinicalMedicine*, 25, 50, 101503.

Anikeeva, O., Brennan, D.S., & Teusner, D.N. (2013). Household income modifies the association of insurance and dental visiting. *BMC Health Serv Res*, 13, 432.

Berglund, E., Westerling, R., & Lytsy, P. (2017). Social and health-related factors associated with refraining from seeking dental care: a cross-sectional population study. *Community Dent Oral Epidemiol*, 45, 258–265.

Bhatti, T., Rana, Z., & Grootendorst, P. (2007). Dental insurance, income and the use of dental care in Canada. *J Can Dent Assoc*, 73(1), 57–57.

Biggs, A. (2012). *Dental Reform: An Overview of Universal Dental Schemes*. Canberra: Parliamentary Library. https://www.researchgate.net/publication/262568389_Dental_reform_an_overview_of_universal_dental_schemes (accessed 13 May 2024).

Blackwell, D.L., Villarroel, M.A., & Norris, T. (2019). Regional variation in private dental coverage and care among dentate adults aged 18–64 in the United States, 2014–2017. *CDC*, 336, 1–8.

Bock, J.O., Hajek, A., Brenner, H. et al. (2017). A longitudinal investigation willingness to pay for health insurance in Germany. *Health Service Res*, 52(3), 1099–1117.

Bock, J.O., Heider, D., Matschinger, H. et al. (2016). Willingness to pay for health insurance among the elderly population in Germany. *Eur J Health Econ*, 17, 149–158.

Brennan, D.S., Anikeeva, O., & Teusner, D.N. (2013). Dental visiting by insurance and oral health impact. *Aust Dent J*, 58, 344–349.

Dror, D.M., Hossain, S.A., Majumdar, A. et al. (2016). What factors affect voluntary uptake of community-based health insurance schemes in low- and middle-income countries? A systematic review and meta-analysis. *PLoS One*, 11(8), e0160479.

Duncan, L. (2014). Effects of income and dental insurance coverage on need for dental care in Canada. *J Can Dent Assoc*, 80, e6.

Eaton, K.A., Ramsdale, M., Leggett, H. et al. (2019). Variations in the provision and cost of oral healthcare in 11 European countries: a case study. *Int Dent J*, 69(2), 130–140.

Footman, K., Kna, I.C., Baeten, R. et al. (2014). *Cross-border Health Care in Europe*. World Health Organization.

Fukuda, K. & Fukuda, Y. (2009). *Cross-border Health Care in the European Union: Recent Trends in Movement of Health Service Professionals, Patients and their Implications*. Bunmadou.

Garla, B.K., Satish, G., Divya, K.T. (2014). Dental insurance: a systematic review. *J Int Soc Prev Community Dent*, 4(Suppl 2), S73–77.

Gnanamanickam, E.S., Teusner, D.N., Arrow, P.G., & Brennan, D.S. (2018). Dental insurance, service use and health outcomes in Australia: a systematic review. *Aust Dent J*, 63(1), 4–13.

Haney, K. (2022). *Does Medicaid Cover Adult Dental Work in Your State*. Growing Family Benefits. https://www.growingfamilybenefits.com/medicaid-cover-dental-work/.

Japanese Australian Support in Community (JASIC) Inc. (2019). *Health care system of Australia* (in Japanese).

Joshua, L. (2017). *Aging and Long-Term Care Systems: A Review of Finance and Governance Arrangements in Europe, North America and Asia-Pacific*. World Bank Group. Discussion Paper, 1705.

Karagiannidou, M., & Wittenberg, R (2022). Social insurance for long-term care. *J Popul Ageing*, 15(2), 557–575.

Kravitz, A.S., Bullock, A., Cowpe, J., et al. (2015). *EU Manual of Dental Practice 2015* (edition 5.1). The Council of European Dentists.

Manski, R.J., Moeller, J.F., & Chen, H. (2014). Dental care coverage and use: modeling limitations and opportunities. *Am J Public Health*, 104(2)e80–e87.

Manski, R., Moeller, J., Chen, H. et al. (2015). Disparity in dental coverage among older adult populations: a comparative analysis across selected European countries and the United States. *Int Dent J*, 65(2), 77–88.

Masters M. (2022). *Dental Coverage Under Original Medicare, eHealth Medicare October 06, 2022*.

Mazevet, M.E., Garyga, V., Pitts, N.B. et al. (2018). The highly controversial payment reform of dentists in France: Seeking a new compromise after the 2017 strike. *Health Policy*, 122(12), 1273–1277.

Mercier, G., Pastor, J., Clément, V. et al. (2019). Out-of-pocket payments, vertical equity and unmet medical needs in France: A national multicenter prospective study on lymphedema. *PLoS One*, 14(5), 1–13.

Ministry of Health, Labour, and Welfare (MHLW) of Japan (2018). Sekaino kouseiroudou 2018, 2017, Kaigaijouseihoukoku (in Japanese). Tokyo: MHLW.

Molarius, A., Simonsson, B., Lindén-Boström, M. et al. (2014). Social inequities in self-reported refraining from health care due to financial reasons in Sweden: health care on equal terms? *BMC Health Serv Res*, 14, 605.

Morgan, S.G., Li, W., Yau, B., & Persaud, N. (2017). Estimated effects of adding universal public coverage of an essential medicines list to existing public drug plans in Canada. *CMAJ*, 189(8)E295–E302.

NHS (2024). *How Much Will I Pay for NHS Treatment?* https://www.nhs.uk/nhs-services/dentists/how-much-will-i-pay-for-nhs-dental-treatment/ (accessed 30 June 2024).

Osterberg, T., Sundh, W., Gustafsson, G., Gröndahl, H.G. (1995). Utilization of dental care after the introduction of the Swedish dental health insurance, *Acta Odontol Scand.*, 53, 349–357.

Pegon-Machat, E., Faulks, D., Eaton, K.A. et al. (2016). The healthcare system and the provision of oral healthcare in EU Member States: France. *Br Dent J*, 220(4), 197–203.

Roberts-Thomson, K.F., & Stewart, J.F. (2003). Access to dental care by young South Australian adults. *Aust Dent J*, 48(3), 169–174.

Ross, J.S. (2002). The committee on the costs of medical care and the history of health insurance in the United States. *Einstein Quart J Biol Med*,19, 129–134.

Saltman, R.B., Busse, R., & Figueras, J. (2004). *Social Health Insurance Systems in Western Europe*. Open University Press.

Schrimshaw, E.W., Siegel, K., Wolfson, N.H. et al. (2011). Insurance-related barriers to accessing dental care among African American adults with oral health symptoms in Harlem, New York City. *Am J Public Health*, 101(8), 1420–1428.

Sinclair, E., Eaton, K.A., Widström, E. (2019). The healthcare systems and provision of oral healthcare in European Union member states. Part 10: comparison of systems and with the United Kingdom. *Br Dent J*, 227(4), 305–310.

Steele, J. (2009). *NHS Dental Services in England*. COI for the Department of Health. sigwales.org/wp-content/uploads/dh_101180.pdf (accessed 13 May 2024).

Steinmo, S., & Watts, J. (1995). It's the institutions, stupid! Why comprehensive national health insurance always fails in America. *J Health Polit Policy Law*, 20(2), 329–371.

Teusner, D.N., Anikeeva, O., & Brennan, D.S. (2014). Self rated dental health and dental insurance: modification by household income. *Health Qual Life Outcomes*, 12, 67.

Teusner, D.N., Brennan, D.S., & Spencer, A.J. (2015). Associations between level of private dental insurance cover and favourable dental visiting by household income. *Aust Dent J*, 60, 479–489.

Thompson, B., Cooney, P., Lawrence, H. et al. (2014). The potential oral health impact of cost barriers to dental care: findings from a Canadian population-based study. *BMC Oral Health*, 14, 78.

Tinker, A. (2003). Ageing in the United Kingdom – what does this mean for dentistry?, *Br Dent J*, 194(7), 369–372.

Tuohy, C.H. (2018). What's Canadian about Medicare? A comparative perspective on health policy. *Healthcare Policy*, 13(4), 11–22.

Willink, A. (2019). The high coverage of dental, vision, and hearing benefits among Medicare Advantage enrollees. *Inquiry*, 56.

World Health Assembly resolution 58.33. (2005). Sustainable health financing, universal coverage and social health insurance. Fifty-eight World Health Assembly.

World Health Organization. (2004). *Tax-based Financing for Health Systems: Options and Experiences.* Geneva: WHO.

World Health Organization. (2014). *Making Fair Choices on the Path to Universal Health Coverage.* Final report of the WHO Consultative Group on Equity and Universal Health Coverage. Geneva: WHO.

World Health Organization. (2019a). *Universal Health Coverage and Health Financing*. Geneva: WHO. https://www.who.int/health_financing/universal_coverage_definition/en/ (accessed 13 May 2024).

World Health Organization (2019b). *Integrated Care for Older People (ICOPE): Guidance for Person-centred Assessment and Pathways in Primary Care, Switzerland*. Geneva: WHO. https://www.who.int/publications/i/item/WHO-FWC-ALC-19.1 (accessed 13 May 2024).

Ziller, S., Eaton, K.E., & Widström, E. (2015). The healthcare system and the provision of oral healthcare in European Union member states. Part 1: Germany. *Br Dent J*, 218, 239–244.

Zivkovic, N., Aldossri, M., Gomaa, N. et al. (2020). Providing dental insurance can positively impact oral health outcomes in Ontario. *BMC Health Serv Res*, 20(1), 124.

6

Health policy in Asia: Overview and vision

Oral Health for an Ageing Population: Evidence, Policy, Practice and Evaluation, First Edition. Kakuhiro Fukai.
© 2025 John Wiley & Sons Ltd. Published 2025 by John Wiley & Sons Ltd.

6.1 Introduction

Ageing is now a global phenomenon that has become an urgent public health challenge all over the world, and it continues to accelerate rapidly. Ageing is a natural biological process which increases the risk of disease, thereby requiring medical care and long-term care (WHO 2015; Asian Development Bank 2022). To confront this challenge, the United Nations (UN) has recommended, as one of its Sustainable Development Goals (SDGs), that universal health coverage (UHC) be adopted in all countries by 2030 (UN 2015). However, there is great variation in the pace at which different countries are progressing toward this goal. With increasing populations and often insufficient resources, most Asian countries are struggling to achieve this goal. It is important for each country to move toward UHC in its own way, depending on the resources it has available.

No matter where one is born in the world, everyone should have equal opportunities, and that includes access to healthcare. In fact, however, health disparities exist both within countries and globally. According to the 2017 Global Monitoring Report issued by the World Health Organization and the World Bank, 'at least half the world's population still lacks access to essential health services. Furthermore, some 800 million people spend more than 10 per cent of their household budget on health care, and almost 100 million people are pushed into extreme poverty each year because of out-of-pocket health expenses' (WHO 2015). Within this context, UHC, which is based on the concept that health is a basic human right, aims to achieve the following goal: 'every individual and community, irrespective of their circumstances, should receive the health services they need without risking financial hardship' (WHO 2015). At a 2019 High-level Meeting of the United Nations, the definition of UHC was further clarified and expanded to include dental health (UN 2019).

In the SDGs adopted at the UN Summit in 2015, the promotion of UHC was included in goal 3 (health and welfare). As of now, the degree of achievement varies in each country and can be categorized into three levels: already achieved; nominally but not functionally achieved; and set as a goal but not yet achieved (El-Jardali et al. 2019).

This chapter represents a close examination of the health insurance systems of Asian countries, which have a large number of elderly people. The characteristics and challenges of the health insurance systems of 10 Asian countries are summarized, with a specific focus on identifying the funding sources of the health insurance system in each country, based on research reports and government records from 2008 to 2018. It is necessary to develop country-specific variations of UHC, and this can best be accomplished by sharing information and incorporating the most useful aspects of each country's system. This process will also contribute to the goal of establishing UHC on a global scale, not only in Asia (Joshua 2017; WHO 2017).

6.2 Rapidly declining birth rate and accelerated ageing in Asia

Population ageing is progressing throughout the world, and Asia is no exception. In 2018, the percentages of the population over 65 in Vietnam and South Korea were 6.7% and 13.0%, respectively, as shown in (The Economist 2018). Vietnam is soon expected to become an ageing society, and South Korea an aged society. The time it takes for the percentage of the population over 65 to double from 7% to 14% is estimated to be 14 years in Vietnam; 16 years in Singapore; 17 years in South

Korea; 19 years in Indonesia; 20 years in Thailand, Malaysia, and the Philippines; and 23 years in China. Over the next 30 years, therefore ageing will accelerate rapidly in Asian countries (Wakabayashi 2006; Masuda and Kim 2015).

Total fertility rate (TFR) has fallen below the population replacement level in many Asian countries, decreasing dramatically from 2.1 to 1.3 in Singapore and falling to 1.5 in Thailand, 1.6 in China, and 2.0 in Malaysia and Vietnam, due to low birth rates (Wakabayashi 2006). A birth rate below population replacement level coupled with accelerated population ageing implies an overall decline in the productive population and therefore the labour force. When this occurs in the early stages of economic development, such as in Thailand or Vietnam, governments must take a two-pronged policy approach, implementing both a social security system for the elderly and a child-care support system for young families at the same time. This poses an impossible financial burden on such governments.

6.3   Funding sources of health insurance systems

Globally, health insurance systems are largely divided into three models: government-funded tax revenue model, the social insurance (multiple-payer) model, and the hybrid model (private insurance combined with tax revenue). The government-funded tax revenue model has been implemented in the UK and other Commonwealth countries like Canada, where the government is the primary provider of medical services, and taxes are the primary financial resource. The social insurance model, characteristic of Germany and Japan, is administered by public (primarily) and private (optionally) insurance organizations that are subsidized to varying degrees by the government but also require payment by service users. The hybrid model, such as that of the US, is when medical insurance for everyone but the poor and elderly is provided by for-profit private companies (Tanaka and Niki 2007).

Health insurance systems in Asia consist of a mixture of the social insurance model and the tax revenue models, providing basic healthcare for those who cannot afford to pay into the insurance system. For example, Malaysia has no public medical insurance system, but it does run a limited number of public hospitals using government funds. The health insurance system in Singapore is referred to as a fund system, where funds are deducted from workers' salaries and saved in individual accounts in a 'Central Provident Fund' for use when healthcare services are required. In countries where the majority of workers occupy the informal labour sector and therefore have unstable incomes, such as Indonesia and India, there is no national health insurance system, so these countries do not fit well into any of the three models described above; however, the resulting reality is that very few citizens have access to healthcare at all. These countries do, however, provide prevention-oriented, community-based health promotion and education activities with government funds (Table 6.1).

Health insurance is often provided for public officials, but rarely for socially vulnerable people such as rural residents, farmers, fishermen, those on a low income and ethnic minorities. In 2008, India adopted a medical health insurance system called Rashtriya Swasthya Bima Yojana (RSBY) for those who are below the poverty line. However, this system only covers certain types of in-patient care while not covering outpatient care or medical products, which comprise most out-of-pocket medical expenses. Some countries, such as Vietnam, have only a small amount of public funding available for healthcare provisions for the poor.

Table 6.1 Funding sources of health insurance systems in Asia.

Country	Insurance scheme	Funding sources			
		Insurance system	Government subsidization	Out-of-pocket payments	Public hospitals
China	Urban Employee Basic Medical Insurance System	+	−	+	−
Urban and Rural Residents' Basic Medical Insurance Systems (formed in 2016)	[Former] Basic Medical Insurance System for Urban Residents	+	+	+	
	[Former] New Rural Co-operative Medical Care System (NRCMCS)		+	−	
India	Central Government Health Scheme (CGHS)	Social insurance system	+		−
	Employees' State Insurance Scheme (ESIS)	Social insurance system	+	−	−
	Rashtriya Swasthya Bima Yojana (RSBY)	−	+	−	
Indonesia	SJSN (System Jaminan Social National) Health	Social insurance system	+	−	Free for the poor
South Korea	Universal health coverage	Social insurance system	+	+	−
Malaysia	No public system of medical health insurance	−	−	+	−
	Private medical facilities with free consultations				
The Philippines	PhilHealth	Social insurance system	+	+	−

Country	Scheme	Type				
Singapore	Medisave	Fund system			−	Partially out-of-pocket
	MediShield	+			+	
	Medifund	−			−	
Thailand	Civil Servant Medical Benefit Scheme (CSMBS)	−	+	−	−	Free for those with low-income
	Social Security Scheme (SSS)	Social insurance system	+	+	+	
	Universal Coverage	−	+		+	
Vietnam	Health Insurance	Social insurance system	+	+	+	−

6.4   Medical health insurance systems in Asian countries

In this section, the characteristics of health insurance systems in Asia are summarized, based on documents from 2008 to 2018 (Table 6.2).

6.4.1   China

China has three medical insurance systems: the Urban Employee Basic Medical Insurance System, the Basic Medical Insurance System for Urban Residents, and the New Rural Co-operative Medical Care System (NRCMCS). The Basic Medical Insurance System for Urban Residents and the NRCMCS are treated separately here, but they were integrated to form the Urban and Rural Residents' Basic Medical Insurance System in 2016 (Chen et al. 2017; Liu et al. 2017; Katayama 2018; MHLW of Japan 2018; Wang et al. 2018).

6.4.1.1   Urban employee basic medical insurance system

This is compulsory coverage for company workers living in the city, including those with both urban and rural family registers, the self-employed, public officers and retired public officers. It is composed of two-storey structure: a personal account (personal savings) and a collective fund (social insurance system). Insured people can visit hospitals for treatment and receive medicine at pharmacies, but clinics are not covered under the medical insurance system. The personal savings accounts cover basic medical expenses such as treatments and medication, while the collective fund covers high-cost examinations, treatments and hospitalization for specific diseases. Both funds draw from the public medical insurance fund.

6.4.1.2   (Former) basic medical insurance system for urban residents

This is optional coverage for the unemployed, the elderly, the disabled, students and children under age 16 with urban family registers.

6.4.1.3   (Former) new rural co-operative medical care system (NRCMCS)

This system was designed to provide optional affordable coverage for rural residents. The new Urban and Rural Residents' Basic Medical Insurance Systems, formed in 2016, has a two-storey structure. Basic medical expenses are covered by the public medical insurance fund, while high-cost examinations, treatments and hospitalization for specific diseases are covered by public–private collaboration.

6.4.2   India

Three medical insurance systems exist in India: the Central Government Health Scheme (CGHS) for public servants, the Employees' State Insurance Scheme (ESIS) for private sector employees, and RSBY for the poor. The poor are defined as households that are below the poverty line as determined by the government. People insured under ESIS and RSBY can access free medical care at registered medical institutions. These medical security systems do not rise to the level of UHC because a very small percentage of the Indian population meets the conditions required to join these systems.

6.4.2.1   Central government health scheme (CGHS)

This system is funded by social insurance and public expenditure. Premiums of 250–1000 rupees per month are paid out of the insured person's salary. Public subsidization is provided from the central government budget. Coverage includes comprehensive medical care such as outpatient care, hospitalization and medicine.

Table 6.2 Health insurance systems in Asia.

Country	Insurance scheme	Legal basis	Year implemented	Administration	Funding sources — Insurance system	Funding sources — Government subsidization	Eligibility	Benefits	Out-of-pocket payments	Number of people covered	Public hospitals
China	Urban Employee Basic Medical Insurance System	Social Insurance Act	Introduced in 1951 Renewed in 1998	Municipal government	First storey (personal accounts for basic medical care) ● Employer burden: total wages of employees × 8% ● Employee burden: average previous year's wage × 2% Second storey (collective fund for high-cost medical care): different in each region	—	Urban employees (city or provincial family register), self-employed, civil servants	First storey: basic medical expenses Second storey: high-cost exams, treatments, hospitalization for specific diseases	Personal account savings are used to pay for medical treatments and medication (public funding for both first and second stories)	295.32 million (2016) Coverage rate: 52.4%	
	Urban and Rural Residents' Basic Medical Insurance System (formed in 2016)	(Former) Basic Medical Insurance System for Urban Residents	Social Insurance Act	2007	Municipal government	First storey (basic medical insurance): users pay by selecting from a number of pre-set premiums, which differ by region Second storey (medical insurance for serious diseases): basically no payment required	Provincial/ district governments subsidize a certain amount for each inhabitant each year	The unemployed, the elderly, the disabled, students and children with urban family registers	First storey: basic medical expenses (covered by public medical insurance fund) Second storey: high-cost exams, treatments and hospitalization for specific diseases (funded by public–private collaboration)	Regulated by local government	448.6 million (2016)	
		(Former) New Rural Co-operative Medical Care System (NRCMCS)	Social Insurance Act	Introduced in 1959 Renewed in 2003	Prefectural and municipal government		Provincial government anually subsidizes over 10 yuan per person	Rural citizens with provincial family registers		Free	670 million (2016) Coverage rate: 98.8%	

(Continued)

Table 6.2 (Continued)

Country	Insurance scheme	Legal basis	Year implemented	Administration	Funding sources			Eligibility	Benefits	Out-of-pocket payments	Number of people covered	Public hospitals
					Insurance system	Government subsidization						
India	Central Government Health Scheme (CGHS)		1954		Social insurance system (salary of an insured persons)	Central government budget		Senior citizens and retired central government personnel	Specialist consultations, hospitalization, pharmaceuticals		2.97 million (2015)	
	Employees' State Insurance Scheme (ESIS)	The Employees' State Insurance Act	1952	Employees' State Insurance Corporation (ESIC)	Social insurance system Employer contribution: 4.75% of employee wages Employee contribution: 1.75% of wages	Provincial government subsidizes 12.5% of medical costs		Private sector employees	Medical services, sickness, maternity (services provided in kind) Allowance for invalidity and funeral expenses (cash payments)	Free	29.3 million (2017)	Free
	Rashtriya Swasthya Bima Yojana (RSBY)		2008	Provincial governments (based on the guidelines of the Ministry of Labour and Employment)	—	Central government: 75% provincial government: 25%		Below poverty line (BPL) Five household members (including the head of the household) are covered	Hospitalization in registered hospitals, 100 rupees hospitalization-related transportation, transportation for screening and monitoring	Free	36 330 households (2017)	

| Indonesia | SJSN (System Jaminan Sosial Nasional) Health | Act on the National Social Security System | 2014 | Badan Penyelenggara Jaminan Sosial (BPJS) | Social insurance system
1) Civil servants, military personnel, and police officers: contribution is 5% of monthly wages. Employers pay 3/5, and employees pay 2/5
2) Other salaried labourers: contribution is 5% of monthly wages. Employers cover 4/5, and employees cover 1/5
3) Non-salaried labourers and the unemployed: contributions differ according to hospital ward and service provided
4) Pensioners: contribution is 5% of basic pension and family allowance. The government covers 3/5 and the pensioner covers 2/5 | The government covers medical care for the poor | Entry obligation for all citizens started on 1 January 2019 All citizens (the poor, employers, labourers); foreigners working over 6 months in Indonesia | Hospitalization, specialist consultation, medication, maternity and emergency treatment | Free Out-of-pocket for expenses that exceed an amount determined by Ministerial Ordinance | 1.27 billion (2014) | Inexpensive medical treatments and medication Free for the poor Subsidized by the central government |

(*Continued*)

Table 6.2 (Continued)

Country	Insurance scheme	Legal basis	Year implemented	Administration	Funding sources		Eligibility	Benefits	Out-of-pocket payments	Number of people covered	Public hospitals
					Insurance system	Government subsidization					
South Korea	Universal health coverage	National Health Insurance Act	1977 1989 (UHC)	National Health Insurance Corporation (NHIC) Health Insurance Review and Assessment Service (HIRA)	Social insurance system Employment-based health insurance: contribution is 5.89% of monthly bonus and 2.945% of monthly salary. Employers and employees contribute equally Community medical insurance: according to an individual's income and assets (2013)	Public revenues General tax and tobacco tax (2012)	All residents of South Korea Divided into three groups: employees, dependents and community members	Medical allowances, medical expenses, allowances for support/mobility equipment for those with disabilities, maternity consultations and medical check-ups	• Hospitalization: 20% • Meals during hospitalization: 50% • Consultations: 30–60% • Medication: 30–50% • Serious conditions: 5% • Incurable conditions: 10%	National Health Insurance: 49.662 million	
Malaysia	No public system of medical health insurance Private medical facilities with free consultations								In 1951, medical treatment fees at public hospitals were set in accordance with the Fees Act. Federal subsidization of public hospitals reduces the out-of-pocket expense for patients.		
The Philippines	PhilHealth	Republic Act No.7875	1995	Philippines Health Insurance Corporation (PHIC) (PhilHealth)	Social insurance system Contribution is 2.5% of an employee's salary. Employers and employees contribute equally	National government provides coverage for indigenous residents Local governments provide coverage for low-income residents	All citizens in the Philippines	Hospitalization, expensive medical treatments, specialist consultation	Hospitalization and medical consultation costs that exceed the amount covered by the government	80.67 million (2013)	

Country	Scheme	Act	Year	Administrator	Funding	System	Eligibility	Coverage	Cost	Enrollment	Notes
Singapore	Medisave	Central Provident Fund Act (Chapter 36)		Central Provident Fund Board	—	Medical savings account system Employers and employees contribute a percentage of the salary to the employee's personal account	Employed citizens, permanent residents, the self-employed (if income exceeds a certain amount) and seamen of foreign nationality	Hospitalization, chronic diseases, expensive exams and allowances for medical expenses	Free	3.42 million (2012)	$20–30 per consultation Available to the general public Reduced treatment fees for those over 65 and children
	MediShield	Central Provident Fund Act (Chapter 36)	2014	Central Provident Fund Board	—	Social insurance scheme Annual insurance fee is set according to age	All Medisave members must join	Hospitalization, chronic diseases, expensive exams and medical costs that exceeds the coverage of Medisave	Costs which exceed the maximum limit of insurance claims, based on length of hospitalization or type of surgery	–	
	Medifund	Medical and Elderly Care Endowment Schemes Act (Chapter 173A)	1993	Medifund Committee	The National Treasury covers all costs	—	Citizens of Singapore	Hospitalization, specialist consultation and nursing care	Free	587,481 (2012)	
Thailand	Civil Servant Medical Benefit Scheme (CSMBS)	Imperial Ordinance	1980	Central Accounting Bureau in Ministry of Finance	Funded by taxes	—	Current and retired public servants in government organizations	All-inclusive coverage (in-kind provision)	Generally free of charge Out-of-pocket: hospitalization in private hospitals	4.97 million (2012) Coverage rate: 8%	30-baht out-of-pocket payment per consultation Free for low-income persons
	Social Security Scheme (SSS)	Social Security Act	1991	Social Security Office in Ministry of Labour	Government subsidization: 2.75% of the employee's wages	Social insurance system Contribution is 10% of an employee's wages; employees and employers split the burden	Compulsory registration: employees of private companies, aged 15–59 Voluntary registration: farmers and the self-employed	Consultations, nursing care, medication, transportation (in-kind) Cash payments also provided	Disability allowance within the social insurance scheme: free consultation within fixed limits	14.04 million (2016) Coverage rate: 21%	

(Continued)

Table 6.2 (Continued)

Country	Insurance scheme	Legal basis	Year implemented	Administration	Funding sources			Benefits	Out-of-pocket payments	Number of people covered	Public hospitals
					Insurance system	Government subsidization	Eligibility				
	Universal coverage	National Health Security Act	2002	National Health Security Office (NHSO)	—	Funded by taxes	Voluntary registration: farmers and the self-employed who are not in CSMBS or SSS	Treatment of acute symptoms (in-kind) Disease prevention activities No cash payments	30-baht payment per consultation/ hospitalization	48.62 million (2012) Coverage rate: 75%	
Vietnam	Health insurance	Health Insurance Act (25/2008/ QH12) Health Insurance Act (46/2014/ QH13)	2009 2015	Ministry of Health (MOH) Viet Nam Social Security (VSS)	Social insurance systems: 1) Employee-employer contributions: employees in private companies and civil servants 2) Unemployent and retirement 3) Voluntary contributions: persons employed in agriculture, forestry and fisheries, and the self-employed	1) Fully subsidized by government: government officials, the poor, minorities in socially and economically difficult situations, children under 6 and their families 2) Partially subsidized by government: students, quasi-low-income residents	Compulsory registration: Contract workers who have worked longer than 3 months, civil servants, occupational accidents and unemployment, the poor, minorities in difficult situations, foreigners who have received a Vietnam government scholarship, children under 6, students, and workers in agriculture, forestry and fisheries	• Consultations, treatments, rehabilitation, regular pre-natal check-ups and childbirth • Hospital transfer costs from lower-level hospital to higher-level one in case of emergency hospitalization, children under 6 and the poor	1) Consultations and treatments are paid for by a combination of the health insurance fund and out-of-pocket payments. The percentage paid from the health insurance fund depends on the category of the insured person (three categories) 2) In case of treatment at inappropriate-level hospital, payment from the health insurance fund will be reduced	64.65 million Coverage rate: 70% (2014)	

6.4.2.2   Employees' state insurance scheme (ESIS)

This system is funded by premiums, and the Employees' State Insurance Corporation (ESIC) is the administrating body. The employer burden amounts to 4.75% of the employee's wages, and the employee burden is 1.75%. Provincial governments subsidize 12.5% of covered medical costs, up to a maximum of 15 000 rupees per person annually. Coverage includes in-kind services such as out-patient care and hospitalization, as well as cash payments such as invalidity allowances.

6.4.2.3   Rashtriya swasthya bima yojana (RSBY)

This system is administered by provincial governments and subsidized by both the central government (75%) and provincial governments (25%). There is no burden imposed on users to pay insurance premiums. At registered medical institutions, the insured can be hospitalized for free surgery and provided with transportation expenses.

The healthcare costs at public hospitals are free thanks to RSBY. However, due to a shortage of medical facilities, long waits for medical services are common (Haddad et al. 2011; Singh et al. 2014; MHLW of Japan 2018; Sood et al. 2018).

6.4.3   Indonesia

Sistem Jaminan Sosial Nasional Health (SJSN Health) was introduced in 2014 and is managed by BPJS (Indonesia's social security administration). Eligibility is extended to all Indonesian people as well as foreigners working in Indonesia for over 6 months. In general, insured people can get medical treatment for free. Funding sources consist of premiums and government subsidization. Insurance premiums vary depending on one's occupation and the type of services offered. The government subsidizes coverage for those living in poverty. Over 30% of citizens were uninsured in 2014, despite the government's aim to achieve UHC (Sparrow et al. 2013; Fujinami et al. 2015; MHLW of Japan 2018).

6.4.4   South Korea

Social health insurance was introduced with the National Health Insurance Act in 1977, which provided coverage for industrial workers in large corporations. It was expanded to include other workers such as public servants and private teachers in 1978, farmers and fishermen in 1988, and urban areas in 1989. This programme achieved UHC in 1989, and registration is compulsory for all residents of South Korea.

It is operated by the National Health Insurance Corporation (NHIC) and the Health Insurance Review and Assessment Service (HIRA). Funding sources consist of premiums which are shared equally by employers and employees, as well as public revenue obtained from general taxes and tobacco taxes (Kang et al. 2009; Lee et al. 2017; MHLW of Japan 2018).

6.4.5   Malaysia

Malaysia is aiming to provide fair access to medical services without implementing a public medical insurance system. Residents can receive medical services at public medical institutions at a low cost due to subsidization from the federal budget. Medical treatment fees at public medical institutions are set according to the Fee Act of 1951. Additional expenses such as examinations, surgery, hospitalization and medicine are provided at a low cost. Private medical institutions, which are concentrated in urban areas, provide medical treatments which are not covered by health insurance (Yu et al. 2008; MHLW of Japan 2018).

6.4.6 Philippines

In 1995, a national healthcare insurance system was established in the Philippines by integrating the medical insurance portions of the Social Security System (SSS) and the Government Service Insurance System (GSIS). The result was the Philippines Health Insurance Corporation (PHIC; also called PhilHealth), which manages nationwide healthcare insurance system but is itself under government control. PhilHealth, headquartered in Manila, has 15 nationwide branches and 72 service facilities. The Philippine government is aiming to develop PhilHealth into a UHC system for all citizens.

Funding sources consist of: (1) social insurance premiums (2.5% of an employee's wages), half of which are paid by employers and half by employees; (2) asset management through investment activities; and (3) public expenditure from the Department of Health and local governments. Insured people receive in-kind benefits mainly consisting of in-patient medical care. The insured can receive care at public and private medical institutions designated by PhilHealth. A portion of medical expenses are reimbursed to physicians and hospitals based on the severity of the illness and the level of the medical facility. PhilHealth does not cover all medical costs incurred by patients at medical institutions. Rather, patients must pay out-of-pocket for medical costs exceeding a certain amount (Kawahara 2008; Tobe et al. 2013; MHLW of Japan 2018).

6.4.7 Singapore

The government in Singapore has not established UHC as a policy goal because it has a very small population and there is a strong belief that individuals must work hard and provide for their own healthcare needs. Government involvement in healthcare is kept at a minimum, providing only indirect assistance.

The medical health insurance system in Singapore is a combination of individual medical savings accounts (this is the primary form of coverage) and a small social insurance scheme as well as a small Medicare-type system. The Central Provident Fund (CPF) operates the medical savings scheme, in which both employers and employees contribute to individual employee savings accounts that can only be used for medical expenses. Overall, there are three medical insurance systems: Medisave, MediShield and Medifund. Patients pay out-of-pocket for outpatient prescriptions and general outpatient treatments such as for colds (Nakata 2008; MHLW of Japan 2018).

6.4.7.1 Medisave

This is a national medical savings scheme operated by CPF, in which individuals are required to save up money in accounts that can be used to pay for healthcare expenses such as personal or family hospitalizations, day surgeries throughout the individual's lifetime, and even after retirement. If not used, the account balance grows and accrues interest.

6.4.7.2 MediShield

This is a health insurance scheme operated by CPF, which helps to pay for certain large and long-term hospital bills without depleting the funds from one's Medisave account. All members of Medisave are required to join MediShield. This health insurance system is subsidized by the government and only applies to medical services at the public hospitals. The benefit is only for the insured person, and the length of hospitalization and types of surgeries covered are limited.

6.4.7.3 Medifund

This is an endowment fund set up by the government and managed by the National Treasury to help low-income people who cannot use Medisave and MediShield to cover the cost of all medical expenses. This coverage is available only for registered members, and it subsidizes the cost of hospitalization, outpatient treatments and nursing care.

As for public hospitals, those in western Singapore are operated by National Health Hospitals (NHG), while Singapore Health (Singhealth) operates those on the eastern side of the country. In case of emergencies, patients are transported to the public hospital in their region. The medical treatment costs, including general outpatient care and prescriptions, are set at a level that ordinary people can afford. Treatment fees are reduced for those over 65 and children.

6.4.8 Thailand

In Thailand, three types of medical insurance are provided by the government: the Civil Servant Medical Benefit Scheme (CSMBS); invalidity benefits provided via the Social Security Scheme (SSS); and universal coverage (UC). In 2002, UC was established, thereby offering access to the public health insurance system to all residents of Thailand. Thailand has therefore achieved UHC (Anutrakulchai et al. 2016; MHLW of Japan 2018).

6.4.8.1 Civil servant medical benefit scheme (CSMBS)

Civil servants who have worked in government organizations have their healthcare needs provided for through the CSMBS. It is funded by tax resources as a form of public welfare. In general, insured people have free choice of medical institutions, and the costs of comprehensive medical care are covered in full. This is an in-kind benefit rather than a reimbursement model.

6.4.8.2 Invalidity benefits of the social security scheme (SSS)

Within the SSS, invalidity benefits are provided for employees in the private sector. It is funded by premiums as well as government subsidies, with employees and employers each shouldering half of the premiums. In general, insured persons can visit medical institutions to which they are pre-registered, and insured people do not need to pay out-of-pocket at the time of consultation, up to a fixed limit. Benefits include both in-kind and reimbursements for services such as consultations, nursing care, medicine and transportation. Payments from the insurer to medical institutions are determined via a capitation payment system.

6.4.8.3 Universal coverage (UC)

Universal coverage, which is funded by tax resources, is based on voluntary registration and is available to all residents, such as farmers and the self-employed, excluding those who are already insured under CSMBS and SSS. In general, insured people can visit only medical institutions to which they are pre-registered (mostly public hospitals). Individuals must pay 30 baht for a consultation, but this fee is waived for those on low incomes. Benefits are in-kind and mainly include treatment for acute symptoms. Payments from the insurer to medical institutions are determined via a capitation payment system.

6.4.8.4 Vietnam

The medical insurance system in Vietnam is managed by the Ministry of Health and Vietnam Social Security (VSS) based on the Health Insurance Act. Eligible people include corporate employees, children, the elderly and workers in agriculture, forestry and fisheries. The insurance coverage rate was about 70% in 2014, despite the government's efforts to achieve UHC. Funding is via a social insurance premium, the amount of which is adjusted depending on the category (there are five categories) of the insured person (Tran et al. 2017; MHLW of Japan 2018).

6.5 Long-term care system in Asia

6.5.1 What is long-term care?

According to the WHO (2022), long-term care consists of personal, social and medical services that help people with declining intrinsic capacity (due to mental or physical disability) maintain their functional ability and dignity, which is their basic human right. Long-term care may be provided by family members, friends or other informal caregivers in the community or by formal caregivers (healthcare professionals). Formal long-term care aims to prevent, mitigate or recover functional decline in older people or others who need it. It can be provided in a variety of settings, such as home care, community-based care, residential care or in a hospital environment. Formal care necessitates outcome assessment using verified checklists and scales such as the frailty scale developed by WHO (2019) in order determine each person's level of dependence and the type of care needed.

6.5.2 Ageing in the Asia-Pacific region

Population ageing is the shift of a country's population distribution towards older people. It is one of the most significant trends facing the world today. This demographic shift is progressing at a faster rate and affecting a larger number of people in the Asia-Pacific region, compared with other global regions, according to the Organization for Economic Co-operation and Development (OECD) and WHO (2020). Between 2020 and 2050, the proportion of the population aged 65 and over is estimated to increase by about 2.5 times in low- and middle-income Asian countries, reaching over 14% for women and 11% for men (Asian Development Bank 2022).

Globally, the number of older people dependent on long-term care is projected to quadruple by 2050. This increase is due to both population ageing (more older people and longer life expectancy) and changing patterns of disability and disease, with an increasing proportion of noncommunicable diseases, which are associated with care dependency. As a result, the increasing demand for long-term care services vis-à-vis their supply is seen as a pressing challenge for Asian countries. That demand has traditionally been offset by cultural norms dictating family support, but if Asian countries follow the urbanization and changing values that characterized economic development in developed countries, they too will need to develop stable long-term care systems.

6.5.3 Increased demand for long-term care: older people living alone

Traditionally, Asian cultures are known to value mutual support among family members, but the data on older people living alone reveals complex differences across global regions. Some Asian countries have high proportions of older people living alone due to the rise of childless couples, which is itself due to changing values, economic pressures and increasing population mobility.

Taking a closer look at the proportion of people aged 65 and over living alone in the various countries and regions of Asia, it has been shown that there are more elderly people living alone in South Korea than in neighbouring countries such as Japan (Hayashi and Komazawa 2022). In East and South-East Asia, the proportion of elderly people living alone is high in many provinces and districts. The differences become even more apparent when the geographical scope is extended to include South Asia, Central Asia and West Asia. The proportion of older people living alone is low in most South Asian countries but high in Iran and Central Asian countries. European countries have very high proportions of older people living alone, while there is great variation among African countries. In other words, the proportion of older people living alone varies from country to country due to the complex interplay of a variety of factors, both cultural and economic.

6.5.4 Long-term care labour supply

The percentage of the workforce engaged in health/medical care and long-term care in each country, based on national census data – 11.9% in Japan, 6.5% in South Korea, 0.5% in Myanmar and 0.2% in Lao PDR – reflect each country's economic development status. It has been reported that there is a shortage of care workers in low- and middle-income countries (Hayashi and Komazawa 2022). Most of these workers are employed in health and medical services, while there is a shortage of social workers, including workers involved in long-term care for older people.

In countries where older people are mostly cared for by family members, occupational categories related to long-term care of older people often do not even exist. For example, in China (including Taiwan and Hong Kong) and Singapore, as well as South Asia, traditional domestic workers become live-in carers when such needs arise. As the population ages, specialised carers emerge and co-exist with health professionals such as nurses, doctors, physiotherapists and occupational therapists. In younger societies, where the need for long-term care is less prevalent, traditional domestic helpers take on the role of long-term care in the home.

6.5.5 Provision of long-term care: nursing homes

Nursing homes are less common in societies where families shoulder most of the burden of care for older people with disabilities. However, even in such societies, care homes for the elderly do exist, providing a residence for older people who cannot live with their families for a variety of reasons. These institutions are maintained by governments (e.g. Vietnam and Japan), religions (e.g. Sri Lanka) or charitable organizations (e.g. Bangladesh) as part of a rudimentary social welfare system. As the number of older people has increased, institutions specializing in long-term care for the elderly have begun emerging (e.g. in China, Japan, South Korea, and other mid- to high-income countries).

6.5.6 Ageing in place

According to an Asian Development Bank (ADB 2022) study, throughout Asia there is a growing preference for older people to remain in their homes ('ageing in place') and communities rather than reside in long-term care facilities. Home- and community-based care programmes that address the need for assistance with daily activities such as dressing and bathing are much more prevalent than residential care, allowing older people to age in their own homes and hometowns. In all countries surveyed, NGOs, community groups and faith-based organizations provide care for older people in their homes and communities, with demand exceeding supply. Residential care is not widely available and is often expensive and therefore not accessible to most of the population.

Where available, publicly funded residential care services often focus on the most basic needs, such as housing and food, rather than specialized geriatric care services.

The family, therefore, remains the bedrock of long-term care in Asia, with the bulk of the responsibility falling on women. However, these traditional patterns of caregiving are under strain due to a variety of forces, including the increased rate of older people dependent on long-term care, labour migration, increased female participation in the workforce and changing social norms. Asian governments tend to place value on maintaining the central role of the family in the provision of long-term care, and some efforts are being made to support families to this end, but such support is still the exception rather than the norm.

In some countries, a cadre of public health volunteers (community health workers) who provide basic health promotion and healthcare also play an important role. In addition, governments have made a number of efforts to encourage the sharing of long-term care responsibilities among multiple service providers.

6.5.7   Toward a sustainable long-term care system

Asia is facing a wave of ageing and therefore needs to find innovative ways to cope with this situation, especially with the increasing demand for long-term care. The family will likely continue to be the backbone of Asian countries' long-term care provisions, but the living arrangements of older people vary considerably, so the long-term care industry needs to be developed further in this region. This requires that governments implement policies to improve the quantity and quality of the care-providing workforce. A family support system that co-exists and interacts with a network of local services is needed. The existing social service infrastructure should be developed further in order to meet the growing need for long-term care (Maharani 2009; Toor and Jindal 2011; Mohd-Dom et al. 2014; Srinarupat et al. 2021; Shin et al. 2021; Cai et al. 2022).

In the end, whether funded by the government or via individual contributions (insurance premiums) or some combination, some form of public long-term care insurance system will eventually be needed in every country in order to meet the needs of rapidly ageing populations.

6.6   Conclusion

The quality and accessibility of health insurance systems vary widely among Asian countries. There are countries where coverage is offered to all or almost all residents, such as in South Korea, Singapore, the Philippines and Indonesia. Countries such as China, India and Vietnam, however, provide very limited coverage for farmers and the self-employed, which make up the majority of their populations. UHC is one solution to this problem. However, there are a number of obstacles preventing many countries from achieving UHC. These include insufficient financial resources, shortage of medical and dental professionals as well as medication and facilities, and the tendency of the wealthy to enrol in private insurance plans. Therefore, it is necessary for each country to work towards achieving UHC in a way that fits with its own specific history and circumstances, while sharing information, advice and successful ideas with each other. This type of cooperation and information sharing can contribute to progress towards achieving UHC not only in Asian countries, but also globally.

While achieving basic UHC should continue to be the priority for Asian countries, these rapidly ageing societies also need to begin providing long-term care services to their citizens. Ageing is proceeding more rapidly in Asia than in the rest of the world, and although most Asian countries have traditionally relied on family caregivers to shoulder the burden of long-term care for older people, changing values surrounding family and work will lead to a rising demand for non-family caregivers and services, as has happened in advanced countries. In response to these needs, Asian countries should begin including a clear long-term care component in UHC-oriented policies and frameworks, even if implementation continues to be limited by economic factors.

References

Anutrakulchai, S., Mairiang, P., Pongskul, C. et al. (2016). Mortality and treatment costs of hospitalized chronic kidney disease patients between the three major health insurance schemes in Thailand, *BMC Health Serv Res*, 16, 528.

Asian Development Bank (ADB) (2022). *The Road to Better Long-Term Care in Asia and the Pacific Building systems of Care and Support for Older Persons*. ADB.

Cai, H., Cheng, Y.T., Ren, X.L. et al. (2022). Recent developments and future directions of oral healthcare system and dental public health system in China in light of the current global emergency. *Sichuan Da Xue Xue Bao Yi Xue Ban*, 53(1), 43–48.

Chen, W., Zhang, Q., Renzaho, A.M.N. et al. (2017). Social health insurance coverage and financial protection among rural-to-urban internal migrants in China: evidence from a nationally representative cross-sectional study. *BMJ Glob Health*, 2, 1–13.

El-Jardali, F., Fadlallah, R., Daouk, A. et al. (2019). Barriers and facilitators to implementation of essential health benefits package within primary health care settings in low-income and middle-income countries: a systematic review. *Int J Health Plann Manage*, 34(1), 15–41.

Fujinami, Y., & Igarashi, K. (2015). Consideration of Indonesian new social security system through the laws. *J Int Health*, 30(2), 103–113.

Haddad, S., Narayana, D., & Mohindra, K.S. (2011). Reducing inequalities in health and access to health care in a rural Indian community: an India-Canada collaborative action research project. *BMC Int Health Human Rights*, 11(suppl 2), S3.

Hayashi, R., Komazawa, O. (eds) (2022). *Health and Long-term Care Information in Ageing Asia*. ERIA Research Project Report, 7. Jakarta: ERIA.

Joshua, L. (2017). *Aging and Long Term Care Systems: A Review of Finance and Governance Arrangements in Europe, North America and Asia-Pacific*. World Bank Group.

Kang, S., You, C.H., Kwon, Y.D., & Oh, E.H. (2009). Effects of supplementary private health insurance on physician visits in Korea. *J Formos Med Assoc*, 108(12), 912–920.

Katayama, Y. (2018). Public medical insurance of China. *Nissei Kiso Ken Report 2018*, 1–13.

Kawahara, K. (2008). Health situations and medical insurance system of Philippines. *Iryo to Syakai*, 18(1), 189–204.

Lee, S.Y., Kim, C.W., Seo, N.K., & Lee, S.E. (2017). Analyzing the historical development and transition of the Korean health care system. *Osong Public Health Res Prospect*, 8(4), 247–254.

Liu, K., Yang, J., & Lu, C. (2017). Is the medical financial assistance program an effective supplement to social health insurance for low-income households in China? A cross-sectional study. *Int J Equity Health*, 16, 138.

Maharani, D.A. (2009). Inequity in dental care utilization in the Indonesian population with a self-assessed need for dental treatment. *Tohoku J Exp Med*, 218(3), 229–39.

Masuda, M., Kim, J.N. (2015). *Social security of Asia*. Horitu Bunka Sya.

Ministry of Health, Labour, and Welfare (MHLW) of Japan. (2018). Sekaino kouseiroudou 2018, 2017, Kaigaijouseihoukoku (in Japanese). Tokyo: MHLW.

Mohd-Dom, T., Ayob, R., Mohd-Nur, A. et al. (2014). Cost analysis of periodontitis management in public sector specialist dental clinics. *BMC Oral Health*, 14, 56.

Nakata, T. (2008) Singapore's healthcare and policy: medicine as a strategy for the nation to survive. *J Health Care Soc*, 18(1), 121–141.

Organization for Economic Co-operation and Development and World Health Organization. (2020) Ageing. In: *Health at a Glance: Asia/Pacific 2020: Measuring Progress Towards Universal Health Coverage*. Paris: OECD Publishing.

Shin, H., Cho, H.A., & Kim, B.R. (2021). Dental expenditure by household income in Korea over the period 2008–2017: a review of the national dental insurance reform. *Int J Environ Res Public Health*, 18(8), 3859.

Singh, A., Purohit, B.M., Masih, N, & Kahndelwal, P.K. (2014). Risk factors for oral diseases among workers with and without dental insurance in a national social security scheme in India. *Int Dent J*, 64, 89–95.

Sood, N., & Wagner, Z. (2018). Social health insurance for the poor: lessons from a health insurance programme in Karnataka, India. *BMJ Glob Health*, 3, 1–6.

Sparrow, R., Suryahadi, A., & Widyanti, W. (2013). Social health insurance for the poor: targeting and impact of Indonesia's Aske skin programme. *Soc Sci Med*, 96, 264–271.

Srinarupat, J., Oshiro, A., Zaitsu, T. et al. (2021). Inequalities in periodontal disease according to insurance schemes in Thailand. *Int J Environ Res Public Health*, 18(11), 5945.

Tanaka, S., & Niki, R. (2007). *Iryouseidokaikaku no kokusaihikaku* (in Japanese). Tokyo: Keiso shobo.

Tobe, M., Stickley, A., del Rosario, R.B., Jr., & Shibuya, K. (2013). Out-of pocket medical expenses for inpatient care among beneficiaries of the National Health Insurance Program in the Philippines. *Health Policy Plan*, 28, 536–548.

Toor, R.S., & Jindal, R. (2011). Dental insurance! Are we ready? *Indian J Dent Res*, 22(1), 144–7.

Tran, B.X., Boggiano, V.L., Nguyen, C.T. et al. (2017). Barriers to accessing and using health insurance cards among methadone maintenance treatment patients in northern Vietnam. *Subst Abuse Treat Prev Policy*, 12, 35.

The Economist (2017). *Pocket World in Figures 2018*. The Economist Pocket Newspaper Ltd.

United Nations (UN) (2015). *Transforming Our World: The 2030 Agenda for Sustainable Development*. https://sustainabledevelopment.un.org/content/documents/21252030%20Agenda%20for%20 Sustainable%20Development%20web.pdf?_gl=1*1r8pzqb*_ga*MTc0MTMxNjI4MS4xNzE1NjAw NTY5*_ga_TK9BQL5X7Z*MTcxNTYyMzIzMi4xLjAuMTcxNTYyMzIzMi4wLjAuMA (accessed 13 May 2024).

United Nations (2019). Political Declaration of the High-level Meeting on Universal Health Coverage "Universal health coverage: moving together to build a healthier world". https://www.un.org/ pga/73/wp-content/uploads/sites/53/2019/07/FINAL-draft-UHC-Political-Declaration.pdf (accessed 13 May 2024).

Wakabayashi, K. (2006). The recent falling birthrate and the aging population issue in East Asia. *Asia Kenkyu*, 52 (2), 95–112.

Wang, Z., Li, X., Chen, M., & Si, L. (2018). Social health insurance, healthcare utilization, and costs in middle-aged and elderly community-dwelling adults in China. *Int J Equity Health*, 17(1), 17.

World Health Organization. (2015). *World Report on Ageing and Health*. Geneva: WHO. https://www. who.int/publications/i/item/9789241565042 (accessed 13 May 2024).

World Health Organization and The World Bank (2017). *Tracking Universal Health Coverage: First Global Monitoring Report*. Geneva: WHO. https://www.who.int/publications/i/item/9789241564977 (accessed 13 May 2024).

World Health Organization (2019). *Integrated Care for Older People (ICOPE): Guidance for Person-centred Assessment and Pathways in Primary Care, Switzerland*. Geneva: WHO. https://www.who.int/publications/i/item/WHO-FWC-ALC-19.1 (accessed 13 May 2024).

World Health Organization (2022). *What Is Long-term Care?* Geneva: WHO. https://www.who.int/europe/news-room/questions-and-answers/item/long-term-care (accessed 13 May 2024).

Yu, C.P., Whynes, D.K., & Sach, T.H. (2008). Equity in health care financing: the case of Malaysia. *Int J Equity Health*, 7, 15.

7

Conclusion: Deploying oral health policy to reduce health injustice in an ageing world

Globally, the population of older people has been growing exponentially. It is predicted that by 2050, 25% of the world's population – around 2 billion people – will be over 60 years old.

The United Nations' (UN) estimates of average life expectancy in various regions of the world show that it is now approaching 65 years in Africa and between 75 and 80 years in Asia, Europe, North America, Latin America and Oceania.

For this reason, many challenges need to be addressed in order to achieve a society in which all older people can live with dignity and security. Such challenges include the establishment and maintenance of a sustainable social security system characterized by comprehensive healthcare provision, a system of long-term care provision, a solid funding base for these services and the continual accumulation of research. The inclusion of dental care coverage in universal healthcare regimes is also an urgent global challenge.

7.1   Global ageing and health

The world population is over 7.79 billion and growing by about 80 million people every year, so we must aim for a society where food, education, housing and healthcare services are provided for this population in terms of their basic human rights. This population growth will continue until 2050–2100, when the global total fertility rate declines to 2.02. Another challenge is global ageing: in 2050, the ageing rate (65 years and over) is projected to be 28% in high-income countries, 22% in upper-middle-income countries, 11% in lower-middle-income countries and 7% in low-income countries (UN 2019). However, the difference between life expectancy and healthy life expectancy varies between 8 and 10 years in all regions of the world. According to the World Health Organization's (WHO) public health framework for healthy ageing (see Chapter 4) (WHO 2015), as people age biologically, they become more susceptible to disease and their risk of frailty increases, as does their risk of developing conditions requiring long-term care. This naturally increases the need to provide healthcare and long-term care services, as well as a barrier-free living environment and social support system, to maintain intrinsic and functional capacities (WHO 2015).

Against the backdrop of these challenges, the 2030 Agenda for Sustainable Development was adopted at the UN Summit in September 2015. The Sustainable Development Goals (SDGs) in that document consist of international targets for the period 2016–2030 in 17 areas, ranging from poverty, hunger and education to climate change and environmental protection (UN 2015). Health-related issues are set out in goal 3, 'Health and well-being for all'. The specific targets most relevant to the field of oral health are: (1) prevention and control of non-communicable diseases (NCDs); and (2) establishment of universal health coverage (UHC), a system where everyone has access to health services at a cost they can afford. The UN defined oral disease as an NCD in a 2011 resolution and specified that oral health coverage should be included in UHC in a 2019 resolution. Although not explicitly stated in the SDGs, oral health is also highly relevant to target (3), population ageing, for reasons that have been detailed extensively in this book.

In a global society where people are increasingly mobile and information is easily shared, local issues become national issues, and national issues become global issues. All countries have limited financial and human resources, but they must take appropriate measures to use those resources to achieve their public health goals. No matter a country's level of economic and social development, we all need to learn from each other's efforts and mistakes as we each strive to improve our own society (Fukai et al. 2017).

The pertinent facts of global oral health are as follows: (1) many oral diseases are preventable; (2) oral diseases have high prevalence and a lifelong impact on people's health; (3) dental and oral health services are still not included in UHC in many countries, which means that, for economic reasons, dental care and preventive services are inadequate; and (4) many oral diseases share common risk factors with NCDs (WHO 2021). An estimated 3.5 billion people worldwide have oral diseases, and according to the Global Burden of Disease Study, untreated dental caries in permanent teeth ranks first in prevalence among all diseases. Severe periodontal disease ranks sixth, untreated dental caries in deciduous teeth ranks tenth, and severe tooth loss ranks 36th (Marcenes et al. 2013). The prevention of oral diseases promotes food intake, communication and social participation, and general health maintenance, which are requirements for maintaining health and well-being throughout one's life. Therefore, the provision of oral health care services is a fundamental human rights issue.

7.2 A rights-based and sustainable oral health monitoring system

Oral disease is consistently prevalent all over the world, regardless of a nation's economic development, and elderly people are particularly susceptible. The global burden of oral disease, therefore, continues to be a serious problem that is often overlooked (Global Burden of Disease Study 2013 Collaborators 2015). As ageing progresses globally, oral health maintenance is now seen not only as a public health issue, but also as a human rights issue, as stated in the Tokyo Declaration (see Chapter 1, Table 1.2). The need for universal access to oral health services is growing rapidly in low-, middle- and high-income countries, but resource availability (including quantity and quality of dental care professionals and facilities, as well as education) varies greatly both within and among countries.

In light of these challenges, international organizations such as WHO and the World Dental Federation (FDI) are encouraging researchers and policymakers to establish monitoring systems in each country (through national dental associations) and share this information globally. By studying such information, each country can carefully plan, implement and improve their own oral healthcare programmes, policies and evaluation frameworks. That information can in turn be shared globally, feeding a continuous improvement cycle.

The global oral health monitoring system envisioned here represents a departure from the unidirectional model, which is characterized by a flow of information from high-income to low- and middle-income countries, proposing instead a multidirectional information-sharing cycle designed to benefit all countries. Such a system is not possible, however, without a globally uniform set of core oral health indicators as well as a global repository for data collection, storage and access. This multidirectional approach, which would allow for natural variation among nations in terms of the pace and method of adoption, is likely to be more efficient in the long term than promoting uniform goals with deadlines that are unachievable by most countries.

Such a monitoring system might be based on the four-step cycle introduced in Chapter 4 (Figure 4.8). Essential to step 1, 'Needs assessment and monitoring', are standardized measurement instruments based on common oral health indicators, which can be based on the FDI's new definition of oral health (Lee et al. 2017): 'Oral health is multi-faceted and includes the ability to speak, smile, smell, taste, touch, chew, swallow and convey a range of emotions through facial expressions with confidence and without pain, discomfort and disease of the craniofacial complex.'

A universal set of core indicators can be used to assess individual and population needs, which is essential for promoting the adoption of oral health policies as well as informing the content of such policies. This is step 2, collaboration between healthcare professionals and policymakers to formulate effective policies and provisions. These are then implemented and/or adjusted in step 3. Step 4 involves continued monitoring and improvement, which are essential for the maintenance of an evidence-driven oral healthcare system that enables people to stay healthy and active while ageing. A cycle with these elements would represent a meaningful step towards reducing both within-country and among-country oral health gaps and towards the creation of an age-friendly world.

7.3 Evidence-based and effective health policy

Evidence generated from health science research is meaningless if it never influences practice and policy. Each country should, therefore, establish a strong and stable cycle that proceeds from research promotion and funding, to evidence accumulation, to local implementation, to national policy (see Chapter 4, Figure 4.1). Evidence can be translated into practice by drawing up and adopting clinical guidelines, initiating health promotion campaigns, and enacting regional or national health policy. Putting evidence into practice at the local level, such as in individual healthcare institutions or communities, is limited in its ability to improve public health at the national level, and in fact can work against it. In his inverse care law, Hart (1971) noted that unhealthy people are less likely than healthy people to access public health programmes. The implication is that when well-intentioned healthcare professionals implement evidence-based care in the absence of a broader regional or national policy, it can result in widening rather than narrowing health inequities, leaving the most vulnerable behind. For this reason, it is of greater importance than most people realize that this process of translating evidence into practice and policy be regionally or nationally implemented and monitored.

Governments must strive to implement *evidence-based* public health programmes and services for two important reasons, both of which stem from the fact that evidence-based practices are likely to be more effective. The first reason is that public health initiatives are expensive, and the expenses are ultimately funded by taxpayers. This means that it is incumbent upon government organizations to implement programmes that are as effective as possible, with an eye not only to improving public health but also to ensuring that public funds are not wasted, thereby yielding a strong return on the investment. The second reason is related to ethics and human rights. Non-evidence-based public health practices carry a greater risk of causing harm to people rather than helping them, and the provision of safe and effective health care is a fundamental human right.

In order to maintain this research–practice–policy cycle, stronger links between researchers and policymakers must be established. Researchers currently have neither the motivation nor the time to inform policymakers of the evidence they have accumulated, while policymakers may have insufficient knowledge of science to be able to translate evidence into policy. Ideally, researchers should polish their communication skills and work harder to communicate their findings in the public sphere, while policymakers should improve their awareness and understanding of scientific evidence. In the meantime, however, there continues to be a great need for science journalists, media commentators and other experts to bridge the gap. Governments also need to fund large-scale health literacy and education initiatives so that citizens can stay informed about high-quality, trustworthy, evidence-based health knowledge.

7.4   Oral health for healthy ageing

Ageing is inevitably accompanied by a decline in the functions of daily living, as well as increasing susceptibility to disease. In terms of oral health as well, tooth loss, declining eating function and reduced saliva output occur with ageing. It is also important to keep in mind that the systemic health effects and oral health effects of ageing have a reciprocal relationship with each other. Particularly salient examples of this phenomenon can be found in the relationship of chewing function with undernutrition/sarcopenia and the association of oral health-related quality of life (QOL) with declining social participation.

Maintenance of dental and oral health is an important predictor of lifelong QOL. Research shows that oral health maintenance helps prevent dental caries, periodontal disease, tooth loss and oral function decline, and this alone contributes to healthy longevity. But maintaining good dental and oral health has also been proven to contribute to the prevention of NCDs, cognitive decline and frailty.

Dental professionals, therefore, contribute not only to oral health maintenance, but also to the prevention of NCDs and frailty, with both of these effects promoting social participation. They do so by delivering preventive care, education and treatment at all stages of life, thereby contributing to the prevention and control of dental caries, periodontal disease, tooth loss and oral function decline. When assessing, diagnosing and treating older adult patients, dental professionals must carefully consider each patient's multimorbidity status and medication regimen, and they also need to assess their patients' physical and mental status. They can then proceed to make an objective assessment of gradual changes in oral function due to ageing (oral frailty). Another imperative when assessing older patients is to improve early detection of oral cancer.

Performing these assessments in outpatient dental clinics is not sufficient to improve the early detection of oral functional decline. Due to the close and bidirectional relationship between oral and systemic health, dental professionals must increasingly maintain close lines of communication with a variety of other healthcare professionals. An effective way to achieve this is to develop comprehensive community healthcare networks that utilize collaborative assessment systems, or at least information-sharing systems, to integrate the efforts of dental clinics, nursing homes and families.

7.5   Concluding remarks

Ageing cannot be stopped, and as society ages, the risk of healthcare-related injustice increases. To combat this, dental professionals must cultivate an increased awareness of social responsibility and their role in contributing to public health.

Population ageing is by no means unique to high-income countries; it is an unavoidable fact for all humans that the risks of disease and disability increase with age. However, establishing and funding systems to maintain the health of older people, including preventing oral diseases and oral function decline, is no easy task. This book is, therefore, intended to help raise the awareness, not only of dental clinicians but also of a wide array of health professionals and policymakers, regarding oral health for an ageing population. It will provide them with the evidence as well as the practical solutions they need to implement effective policies and practices.

References

Fukai, K., Ogawa, H., Hescot, P. (2017, September). Oral health for healthy longevity in an ageing society: maintaining momentum and moving forward. *Int Dent J*, 67(2), 3–6.

Global Burden of Disease Study 2013 Collaborators Global. (2015). Regional and national incidence, prevalence, and years lived with disability for 301 acute and chronic diseases and injuries in 188 countries, 1990–2013: a systematic analysis for the Global Burden of Disease Study 2013. *Lancet*, 386, 743–800.

Lee, J.Y., Watt, R.G., Williams, D.M. et al. (2017). A new definition for oral health. *J Dent Res*, 96, 125–127.

Marcenes, W., Kassebaum, N.J., Bernabé, E. et al. (2013). Global burden of oral conditions in 1990–2010: a systematic analysis. *J Dent Res*, 92(7), 592–597.

United Nations. (2015). *Transforming Our World: The 2030 Agenda For Sustainable Development.* https://sustainabledevelopment.un.org/content/documents/21252030%20Agenda%20for%20 Sustainable%20Development%20web.pdf (accessed 13 May 2024).

United Nations. (2019). *World Population Prospects, The 2019 Revision.* UN.

World Health Organization. (2015). *World Report on Ageing and Health.* Geneva: WHO.

World Health Organization. (2023). *Oral Health: Key Facts.* https://www.who.int/news-room/ fact-sheets/detail/oral-health (accessed 13 May 2024).

Index

Oral Health for an Ageing Population: Evidence, Policy, Practice and Evaluation, First Edition. Kakuhiro Fukai.
© 2025 John Wiley & Sons Ltd. Published 2025 by John Wiley & Sons Ltd.